I0126513

Body-Mind Rejuvenation

An Integrated Step-by-Step Journey to Natural
Prevention, Recovery and Body-Mind Rejuvenation

Dr Vesna Grubacevic, PhD
Nevenka Malic
Chef & Clinical Nutritionist

First published in 2024 by Vesna Corporation Pty Ltd
Level 27, 101 Collins Street, Melbourne, Australia

Copyright
© 2024, Vesna Corporation Pty Ltd, Nevenka Malic and Dr
Vesna Grubacevic

All rights reserved. No part of this book may be copied,
reproduced, adapted, stored in a retrieval system,
communicated or transmitted in any form or by any means
without prior written permission from the authors/publisher.
All inquiries should be made to the authors/publisher at the
address above.

Cover photo by Satyajit Dey on Unsplash; Chapter 14 photo by
David Clode on Unsplash

Author photos taken by Dr Vesna Grubacevic (for Nevenka's
headshot) and John Weninger (for Dr Vesna's headshot)

Recipe photos taken by Dr Vesna Grubacevic

Table of Contents

Dedication

Nevenka's Dedication

I would like to express my gratitude and thanks to my father and grandmother for their wisdom, and to everyone who was there to support me, and steer me in the right direction during the most difficult times of my life. Specifically, I would like to thank my daughter, Vesna, for all her support, the loving care she has given me, and who continues to be there for me. This book is dedicated to my daughter, Vesna, and to everyone who has supported me on my life's journey.

Dr Vesna's Dedication

I would like to thank Nevenka, for so generously donating her knowledge, expertise and tips in this book, and for sharing her life journey to inspire more people to improve their health and wellbeing. I am honoured to be able to co-author such an empowering book with my inspirational mum, best friend, mentor and role model.

Nevenka and I are both passionate about mind-body health, and helping people to be mentally, emotionally and physically healthy. It is a real privilege to contribute to this book, and to share Nevenka's knowledge and experience with you, the reader. This book is dedicated to you, the reader, for having the curiousity and open mindedness to explore natural ways to master your health and wellbeing.

As part of our commitment to giving back, all profits from this book are being donated to fund scholarships to those most in need of mind-body health support.

Disclaimer

The material in this publication is of the nature of general comment only, and does not represent professional or medical advice. It is not intended to provide specific guidance for particular circumstances and it should not be relied on as the basis for any decision to take action or not take action on any matter which it covers. Examples stated in this book are examples only and should not be relied upon. No part of this book may be taken as advice to be relied on in any circumstances whatsoever. **Readers should obtain professional and medical advice where appropriate and/or necessary, before making any such decision.** All liability is hereby expressly excluded in respect of any loss or damage which may arise in connection with the use of or reliance upon any materials and information contained in this publication.

Preface

This is a very special book. It is both a guide to optimal health and wellbeing, as well as an inspiring journey from a beautiful soul – Nevenka Malic.

Nevenka was born and grew up in Croatia under the foothills of the pine forest mountain, Sveta Gora, on the border of Slovenia. She grew up in a family of two brothers and one sister. The Second World War had just ended, life was a challenge and every day was a gift of survival. People were living in a very small community. As a child, she learnt to survive in poverty, every little thing was appreciated. People were living a very simple life in a tight community supporting each other. They were happy as long as they were healthy, and had food to feed the family. You hardly ever heard anyone complain about a difficult life. Because regardless how hard it was, it was a lot better than during the war that had just ended, end of May 1945.

Children didn't have bedtime book stories. Instead, they were told stories that were too frightening to hear - how hard it was during the war and many years afterwards. There was fear in the community of getting into trouble if they spoke up about the government. It was a hard life under communism. Every day people would witness abuse, killing and harassment of poor innocent people because they just didn't do what they were told to do. As a child, Nevenka did not understand what was happening, and was not allowed to ask any questions.

After she finished high school, Nevenka went to Ljubljana, the capital of Slovenia. There she went to a Gastronomy school to study for the Hotel and Restaurant Management Diploma. Later she moved to Croatia, where Nevenka was living in a one-bedroom unit; it was very small and tight for four people. Nevenka decided to sell everything, and bought a one-way air ticket for her family to go to Melbourne.

Nevenka immigrated to Australia with her immediate family at the age of 28; leaving behind extended family, friends and everything that she worked hard for, for over 11 years. With her she brought only personal possessions that fitted into two suitcases. With Nevenka's love of working with food and interest in people, her dream when arriving in Australia was to have her own restaurant.

Arriving in Australia was extremely difficult because she didn't know how to speak or write English. She needed to learn very quickly because of a new culture and living situation. It was also very hard to find a job without knowing how to write or read English. Nevenka also had the added pressure and persistent trauma of dealing with an abusive, alcoholic husband.

As a result, Nevenka didn't have any choice than to take the lowest paid job in the factory until she learnt basic English to be able to communicate with people. While working at a shoe factory, Nevenka taught herself English from a little dictionary that she brought with her from Croatia. During lunch time, the other workers would go out for lunch, while Nevenka had her lunch at work. She brought her lunch from home because she could not afford to buy meals out. While having her lunch, Nevenka would read from her little dictionary. Many times she would be so focused on the English words she was reading that, without realizing it, she had finished her sandwich and was biting her fingers.

Nevenka worked very hard to put food on the table for her family, working long hours to make ends meet. The first five years were the most difficult because of a lack of support with learning English for immigrants in her local area. Six years later, Nevenka learned to confidently speak and write English, and she started working in the hospitality industry, doing what she loves.

Nevenka is grateful to her brother's friends that helped her with furniture that they didn't need any longer; that support was priceless to her. There were many hurdles to overcome, and many times Nevenka asked herself when will life start to get better. With persistence and hard work, in just 8 years Nevenka achieved her dream of owning her own restaurant. That hard work and persistence show that anyone can make their life as they desire. Nevenka was now able to appreciate the good life for years to come. Those times will forever stay with Nevenka to remind her to be grateful for every little thing that life gives, and to appreciate good health.

To achieve her big goal to have her own restaurant business, she took two part-time jobs: in one restaurant as a chef, and in the other as a waitress. She needed to learn as much as possible to see if she could run a restaurant business. After one year, an opportunity presented itself with one of the restaurants where she worked being for sale. Nevenka met with her bank manager to see how she could get a loan.

She could not believe that six weeks later, she was the owner of her own restaurant. She was so excited. Every day was rewarding, she was in her element doing what she is meant to do. She met so many wonderful people during her time in her restaurant. Regardless of the challenges she had, it made her stronger and more determined to pursue her passion in the hospitality industry.

The biggest challenges that she faced as a woman in business were being bullied by men. The men who worked for her were disrespectful; it was hard for men to accept a female boss. Nevenka needed to stand up for herself and on many occasions, she was forced to let some of them go. Then another challenge she faced was with her male competitors who used every trick to try to get her out of her business. She wasn't going to allow anyone to take away all her hard work, and what she had achieved. Nevenka faced so many obstacles in her life (including abuse and trauma since childhood), and thought this is just another one to overcome.

It took many years for women to start to get some respect at the work place. While things are improving, there is still a long way to go for both women and men to have the same respect and opportunities.

After experiencing emotional, psychological, financial and physical abuse and seeking help through the legal system, Nevenka appreciates from her experience why so many people feel let down by the legal system. After her sense of self was crumbled into a thousand pieces, and when she needed the most support to put the pieces together and be able to trust in people and society again, she was let down. She sought support and protection from her daughter, Vesna.

Through all the abuse, trauma and stress Nevenka also developed a number of health issues, including cancer. In this book, Nevenka shares her journey of recovery from major health issues.

In Chapter 1 of this book, Dr Vesna has the honour of educating you, the reader, about the mind-body connection, and how mastering your thoughts, emotions, beliefs and your environment can master your health and wellbeing.

In the subsequent chapters of this book, Nevenka shares her journey of overcoming numerous personal, professional and health obstacles in her life. In addition to inspiring you with her journey, Nevenka also draws on her wealth of experience, knowledge and qualifications to empower you to naturally prevent, recover and rejuvenate your body-mind for optimal health and wellbeing.

Drawing on her qualifications and experience as a Chef, Clinical Nutritionist and health practitioner, Nevenka also shares some of her favourite healthy and nutritious recipes. She created these specifically for her healing journey. This truly is an integrated step by step journey to body-mind rejuvenation.

Chapter 1

Mind-Body Connection & How Your Mind Affects Your Health

Have you ever wondered how your mind affects your body? Would you like to understand the link between your thoughts, emotions, beliefs, stress and your physical health?

1   What is the Mind-Body Connection?

The mind and body are interconnected. Our emotional and mental health is intimately connected to our physical health. This relationship is often referred to as the mind-body connection.   You would have experienced the mind-body connection if you ever thought of public speaking, then you physically felt nauseous or had butterflies in your stomach. Your thoughts affected you physically.

Likewise, if you are sitting upright and looking straight ahead, you are more likely to have positive thoughts and to feel positive emotions. In contrast, if you are slouching in your chair and looking down at the floor, you are more likely to think negative thoughts and have negative feelings. If you constantly worry or stress about work, relationships or life, this can cause physical conditions like muscle tension, headaches, stomach problems and pain.

Your imagination is very powerful. Research has shown that the mind is unable to distinguish between what is real and what is imagined. For example, if you remember a funny memory, you will most likely start to smile or laugh even when there is nothing funny there now. If you remember a scary scene from a movie, your breathing will likely get faster even though there is nothing scary there in your environment now. Simply thinking about a memory or imagining something, will affect how you feel and your physiology. We call this the mind–body connection.

There is an abundance of research proving the mind-body connection. In 1986, Dr Deepak Chopra wrote the book, *Quantum Healing*, and in it he noted that neuro-transmitter bathes every single cell of the body, and that "our cells are constantly eavesdropping on our thoughts and being changed by them." Our internal dialogue or self-talk acts as a suggestion to the unconscious mind. Hence, every thought we have, whether positive or negative, affects every single cell in our body. That is the mind-body connection.

2 How Your Thoughts Affect Your Behaviour and Your Health

Your thoughts are critical in our quantum world. Our thoughts create our reality through our action or inaction. An April 2023 study by researchers at Washington University School of Medicine in St. Louis, showed that "the link between body and mind is embedded in the structure of our brains, and expressed in our physiology, movements, behavior and thinking".

We are constantly programming ourselves. Every time you speak, every thought you have, each emotion you feel, you are either programming yourself for success or failure. This is because these words and thoughts act as direct suggestions to your mind. Every thought you have affects how you feel, which in turn affects your behaviour.

For example, when you are thinking that an activity will be difficult, you probably dread doing it or worry about getting it done. As a result, you put off doing it. In contrast, when you are thinking and expecting that an activity will be fun and easy, you probably feel motivated to do it and you do it with ease.

We are hypnotising ourselves daily with our self-talk. Your self-talk is self-hypnosis. You are putting yourself into a negative hypnotic trance when your words, thoughts, and emotions are negative, and into a positive hypnotic trance when your words, thoughts, and emotions are positive.

For most people, if their thoughts, words, and emotions are negative, generally they are hypnotising themselves to fail. In contrast, if their thoughts, words, and emotions are positive, generally they are hypnotising themselves to succeed.

Our thoughts are linked with a certain feeling (e.g. confidence, happiness, motivation, sadness) and with our posture (i.e. how we sit and stand). For example, as we think about achieving our goal weight, we may be imagining ourselves standing tall, and feeling confident and comfortable in smaller sized clothes. In turn, this will motivate us to change any eating and exercise habits, and to take action to reach our goal weight.

In contrast, as we think about achieving our goal weight, if we feel dread about exercise, or feel apathetic about eating healthy, or think it will be hard, this will demotivate us to make the necessary changes and take action towards our goal. Hence, we will need to change how we think and feel about health in order to be motivated, and achieve our desired health.

All of this (our thoughts, feelings, and posture) affects our behaviour, and our health. It is really important to realise that health is an internal process, and we have influence over it. By taking responsibility for our thoughts, feelings, beliefs, habits, lifestyle, etc., we also take responsibility for making the necessary changes for improving our health.

3   Emotions and Your Health

Emotions are feelings and our way of knowing that something feels comfortable or uncomfortable for us. Research demonstrates that feelings are caused by chemical reactions in our body and brain. Our feelings are, therefore, real rather than imagined. Paying attention to our emotions is very important.

All emotions are good, because they provide us with feedback as to whether something sits well with us or not. Emotions are our friend because they help us to fully experience life. We have dozens of different emotions. Some are positive and empower us to feel, think, and act in positive ways. Examples of positive emotions include: happiness, fun, excitement, peace, determination, confidence, and motivation.

Emotions become your foe when they hold you back from being, doing, and having what you want in life, and when they sabotage your health, relationships, confidence and your success. Examples of negative emotions include: fear, hurt, anger, rejection, guilt, sadness, betrayal and anxiety. Chapter 3 of *Stop Sabotaging Your Confidence* book discusses emotions in much more detail.

We have dozens of different emotions; fear is one of them. Some fear is appropriate in certain situations. When our fear "buttons" are pushed and we feel overwhelming fear or when we react to a person or situation in a way that we are unhappy with, then fear is out of proportion. Out of proportion fear causes indecision, inaction, avoidance, distraction and procrastination.

Our fears also become self-fulfilling. After a while, we attract what we fear; our thoughts affect our behaviour. For example, people who fear rejection often say or do things to sabotage themselves. In turn, they are rejected.

While all emotions are good, if we hold onto negative emotions for too long and they remain out of proportion, they can create negative effects for our health and overall well-being. One of the negative consequences of suppressing or ignoring our emotions is poor health. There is much scientific research showing the link between negative emotions, and our health and well-being.

According to research at Concordia University, for instance, harbouring bitterness for a long time can result in anger. In turn, if strong enough, this can affect physical health (including the metabolism, the immune system, and organ function). A 2013 study at Ohio University demonstrated that dwelling on negative events can increase inflammation levels in the body. Another piece of research at Ohio State University in 2013 demonstrated that loneliness negatively affects the immune system by increasing inflammation in the body.

A 2014 study published in the *European Heart Journal*, found that "in the two hours immediately after an angry outburst, a person's risk of a heart attack (myocardial infarction (MI) or acute coronary syndrome (ACS)) increased nearly five-fold

(4.74%), the risk of stroke increased more than three-fold (3.62%), and the risk of ventricular arrhythmia also increased compared to other times when they were not angry. The researchers found that the absolute risk increased if people had existing risk factors such as a previous history of cardiovascular problems, and the more frequently they were angry."

In 2016, a 20-year study at the University of California, Berkeley, and Northwestern University published in the journal *Emotion*, showed "... a new level of precision in how emotions are linked to health, and how our behaviors over time can predict the development of negative health outcomes." Further, this study discovered that "The spouses who were observed during their conversations to fly off the handle more easily were at greater risk of developing chest pain, high blood pressure and other cardiovascular problems over time. Alternately, those who stonewalled by barely speaking and avoiding eye contact were more likely to develop backaches, stiff necks or joints and general muscle tension."

If negative emotions are left unaddressed for too long, they can weaken the body's immune system. In turn, this can increase the likelihood of colds, flus, infections and other health issues. Further, when we are feeling negative emotions, we may be less motivated to take care of our health. For example, we may not feel like exercising, eating nutritious foods, etc. Emotional eating and addictions to substances can also be developed as a result of suppressing our emotions, and not addressing the negative emotions.

Given the possible negative impacts of negative emotions, it is important to address any out-of-proportion fears and other emotions to improve our motivation, confidence, health and well-being.

4   Beliefs and Your Health

Beliefs are what we wholeheartedly believe: what we know to be true about ourselves, our self-image, our abilities, our health, other people, and the world around us. Beliefs are our convictions about what is possible, what we can or cannot do, and what we accept as true.

While many of our beliefs were developed during our childhood, early schooling, and early adult life, they can significantly impact on our health and wellbeing today. Like emotions, our beliefs are stored at the unconscious level. Chapter 4 of *Stop Sabotaging Your Confidence* book discusses beliefs in much more detail.

Beliefs determine our reality. If our beliefs are positive (e.g. I am a healthy person) they support us in creating good health. If our beliefs are limiting (e.g. I can't be healthy) then these can limit our ability to be healthy. Whatever we believe, whether positive or negative, becomes real, because it affects our thoughts, feelings, and behaviour, and how we respond to people and situations.

Beliefs are critical to a person's health. Dr Deepak Chopra and many other medical doctors have witnessed terminal patients making a full recovery because of having a belief contrary to their diagnosis. After many experiences with his patients, in the book *Love, Medicine, and Miracles*, Siegel notes that almost all disease originates to some extent in the mind. Hence, the importance of letting go of any limiting beliefs to heal ourselves, and to live healthy lives.

There are different types of beliefs that can impact on our health:

Cultural beliefs

These are beliefs imposed by society e.g. fear of illness. Fears shared with others of our culture can affect us significantly because our fears can become self-fulfilling. In the 19th century fear of tuberculosis (TB) was high, and killed many thousands of people.

Once Dr Robert Koch discovered in 1882 that the cause of TB was a bacterium and this was made known to the general public, death rates from TB dropped significantly despite the absence of an effective drug treatment for the illness for another 50 years. The mystery as to the cause of the illness was solved and, hence, reduced the fear. Cultural beliefs and fears can be changed with educational programs.

Beliefs about our attitude

Research has shown that pessimists get more colds than optimists. Pessimists tend to stress more, and stress lowers the immune response.

Unconscious beliefs

Deep convictions about ourselves e.g. I am not good enough, I can't succeed, I am fat, I don't fit in, etc. These limiting beliefs lead to negative self talk, which causes us to feel negative emotions about ourselves.   In turn, these sabotage our behaviour. For example, if we wish to lose weight, the belief "I am not good enough" can sabotage our motivation, and any changes we wish to make to our eating and exercise habits.

Beliefs about our faith/spiritual beliefs

If we believe we need to be punished for our wrong doing, sometimes that self-talk becomes an unconscious suggestion to create ill health.   Our unconscious mind can accept both positive and negative suggestions without question. Then when people have ill health, they reinforce that belief by saying something like "I am being punished".

Beliefs about an illness

A 2012 study showed that how a person views their illness may be more important to their health outcome than the severity of the illness. Our beliefs about an illness, how it was caused, the duration of the illness, the impact on our family/career/life, the effectiveness of treatment, etc. all impact on our ability to recover and get well.   The study adds that "patients' perceptions of their illness guide their decisions about health", and that treatments need to consider the patient's perceptions for best recovery and success.

Prestige suggestion beliefs

When we hold people like doctors and practitioners in high regard, respect their advice, and we act upon their advice without second thought, this is a prestige suggestion in hypnosis.   That means that the diagnoses and suggestions offered by doctors and other practitioners, are acted upon without question by their patients.

If a negative suggestion is made, accepted and believed by patients as true, it can negatively impact on their health. Also the beliefs and attitudes of doctors and other practitioners towards their patients and their ability to heal and get well, can impact patients' beliefs about their ability to heal, their recovery time, etc.

By changing our beliefs, we can change our self talk, emotions, behaviours and habits, and hence improve our health.

5   Stress and Your Health

Stress is the reaction people have when faced with a stressor. A stressor is a situation or event that causes physiological and/or psychological strain or requires that a major adjustment be made by the individual. Examples of stressors include: conflict, change in health/finances/lifestyle, change in responsibilities, pressure to perform, separation, divorce, job loss, retrenchment, illness, death in the family, etc.

Regardless of the stressor, how you relate to or interpret your environment will determine whether something is stressful to you or not. This varies from person to person.

Dr. Siani argues that it isn't the stressful situations themselves that cause stress, "it's our way of reacting to the situations that makes a difference in our susceptibility to illness and our overall well-being... Instead of discharging this stress, however, we hold it inside where its effects become cumulative..... when chronic stress goes unreleased, it suppresses the body's immune system and ultimately manifests as illness." Therefore, anything that produces the relaxation response and assists us in releasing unresolved emotions, etc. is effective in improving functioning of the immune system, and increasing our defences against illness and disease.

Constant or ongoing stress can lead to chronic stress, which affects the cells in our body. This has the mind-body focused on survival, which can affect our decision-making, problem solving and creativity. When people are stressed, they heal more slowly and their lifespan can be reduced.

Stress can impact all the major mind-body systems, and this varies from person to person:

- Central nervous system: headaches, depression, sleep problems
- Immune system is reduced, inflammation is increased
- Digestive system: appetite, stomach pain/discomfort, heartburn, ulcers, irritable bowel, leaky gut
- Reproductive system: libido, intimacy, increased premenstrual pain, difficulty conceiving
- Musculoskeletal system: lower back pain, chronic pain
- Cardiovascular system: high blood pressure, heart attack, stroke, inflammation
- Endocrine system: abdomen fat accumulation, reduced insulin sensitivity
- Respiratory system: shortness of breath, rapid breaking

According to Dr Lipton, "Almost every major illness that people acquire has been linked to chronic stress. Between 75 and 90 percent of primary-care physician visits have stress as a major contributing factor."

Different people have different coping strategies for dealing with stressors, as well as different thresholds or tolerance levels to stress. Some people lack coping strategies or have low thresholds, and are much more easily stressed by situations that others find easy to deal with. It is important to have coping strategies for stress otherwise stress can adversely affect our wellbeing, and can lead to more serious health problems e.g., anxiety, depression, illness.

6 The Power of Suggestion

We are subject to programming on a regular basis, which acts as a suggestion. Examples include: the ideal body shape and weight we should be is suggested in magazines, what happy couples do, buy and look like on television ads, etc. Some people are more suggestible to these than others.

The most suggestible are babies and young children because they lack the ability to think logically. This is because their critical faculty, the ability to think logically, develops from about age five or six. From then on, they can choose what to believe, and what to ignore. Their critical faculty is at play, and for any information to reach the unconscious mind it must bypass their critical faculty.

Any suggestions are much more powerful and more quickly accepted when emotions are involved. For example, repeated suggestions that induce a fear response are quickly accepted through repetition.

Prestige suggestions are also more powerful as we act upon those suggestions without question because we respect and believe the authority of the source of those suggestions e.g.

doctors, teachers, parents. This is where the placebo and nocebo effects play a key role.

Placebo effect

This is where the patient holds a positive belief that they are getting a helpful drug or treatment, and instead they are getting no actual drug/treatment. For example, if the patient believes that they are receiving a helpful drug and they only receive a sugar pill, this will result in the same therapeutic effect as if the actual drug had been given to the patient.

Nocebo effect

This is where the patient holds a negative belief and expectation that the drug or treatment will cause harm. Hence, that belief and expectation can result in that negative effect to their health. Even statistics of survival from an illness or disease act as a nocebo if the patient believes in and puts themselves in the low survival category.

The Media

The media understands the power of suggestion. The average person spends the equivalent of about 15 years of their life in front of the television, and puts much faith in what they hear, see and feel as they watch television. Advertising is also constantly making suggestions to us, about how to look, what to wear, what to buy, what health, happiness and success look like, etc.

By watching television, listening to the radio, reading magazines/news, we are subjecting ourselves to a myriad of suggestions which are potentially creating our patterns of thinking, feeling, habits and health. Over the past 23 years, I have been cautioning clients about watching the news. Unfortunately, the news is biased to the negative, and much good news is ignored and goes unreported. I call it national depression hour because it is all negative. Notice how you feel after you watch the news.

Other environmental influences

The science of epigenetics explains how mechanisms other than changes in the underlying DNA sequence (e.g. our environment and our life experiences) affect our genetic activity. The cells that make up our whole mind-body are influenced by our environment, so we need to choose our environmental influences carefully.

Negative suggestions by others regarding health need to be avoided. For example, family and friends talking about a history of x illness in the family becomes a suggestion to also have that illness because you are part of the same family. Yet, not everyone in the same family will have the same illness because of lifestyle and so many other factors discussed above.

According to the Cancer Council Victoria website, "only a small percentage of certain cancers (up to 5%) are due to an inherited faulty gene. A faulty gene increases the risk of cancer, but it does not mean every family member will develop the disease." They also cite lifestyle as major contributors to cancer risk, and making lifestyle changes being important to preventing cancers. Instead of blaming your genes for your health, change your lifestyle to improve your health.

The most powerful suggestions

By far the most powerful suggestions are the ones we give to ourselves via our self talk. If our self talk is positive, it has a positive effect on our health.   If it is negative, it has a detrimental effect on our health. Even the words we speak out aloud impact on our health. This is where the notion of organ language comes into play. For example, if you say to yourself "that is a pain in the neck" often enough, after a while your unconscious mind will act upon that suggestion and create a physical pain in your neck. This is because the unconscious mind is unable to analyse, and literally accepts all your suggestions.

This is why it is so important to address all your unresolved past emotions, limiting beliefs, and deeper core issues. For as long as these are left unresolved, they will create negative self talk. In turn, this will sabotage your behaviour and healthy habits, and impact negatively on your health.

7   Keys to a Healthy Mind-Body

The most important step to a healthy mind-body is to take personal responsibility for your own health, rather than relying on anyone else to heal you. After all, all healing is self healing! We heal ourselves, no one else can heal us. This is because only we are in control of how we think, feel, our habits, our behaviours, and therefore our health and life.

It is also important to have a holistic approach to our health. This includes:
- Spiritual: clarity of purpose and direction in life

- Mental: goals and dreams, and focusing on what we want
- Emotional: addressing negative emotions, limiting beliefs and deeper core issues
- Physical: taking enough appropriate action to support the above, including our eating and exercise habits, environment, nutrition, lifestyle, etc.

Because stress is a major contributor to illness and disease, working on the emotional level is critical for a healthy mind-body. This in turn then supports our spiritual, mental and physical wellbeing too. We gain greater clarity of purpose when our fears, anxieties, self-doubts and deeper core issues are addressed. We find it easier to know what we want/our goals, and to focus on what we want. We also find it much easier to change our environment, health and lifestyle habits and behaviours to support optimal health.

You will find additional resources to empower you for optimal mind-body health in the Appendix at the back of this book.

Enjoy reading the subsequent chapters of this book which delve into more detail on achieving optimal mental, emotional and physical health. Those are written from Nevenka's first person perspective as she shares her personal life and health journey, keys to optimal health, and her favourite healthy and nutritious recipes, with you.

Chapter 2
Food Was Our Medicine!

When I take myself back in time, simply observing how many things are taken for granted and wasted today, it gives me a different perspective of life that I lived as a child. Back then in my time as a child, food was very simple. Everything came from the land, except salt and sugar which we used in very small amounts. Food was prepared by season, and everything was grown organically. There was no knowledge of any chemicals until 1955, at least not in the outskirts of the big cities.

This started to change in the late 1950's. Well-off farmers were able to afford to purchase chemical fertilizers to produce a bigger yield of crops. I remember it well. The attitude of arrogance started to spread amongst the well to do farmers, and to suppress poor farmers who fought for survival and to feed their families.

That attitude started to affect the children at school, with competition about whose lunch was better. Children from poor farmers continued to bring whole meal bread and "poor man" food to school. At the same time, children from well-off farmers brought pure white bread and cakes, and teased us as to how poor we were. They forgot that not long ago they were eating the same food as us.

In school we were taught how to keep hygiene. Before each break, we needed to stand in line to wash our hands, sit at our desk, place our napkin/tea towel on the desk, and put our food on it. When we finished eating, we needed to fold our napkin, and put it in our bag for the next day. We needed to carry a handkerchief in our pocket to use in case we sneezed. Children needed to come to school clean, clothing ironed, and hair brushed (if girls had long hair it needed to be tied back into a pony tail or in a plait). There was no such thing as boys with long hair. We were educated for the future, for the time when we were ready to go to the city for higher education. This was valuable knowledge to gain at an early age which would serve us for the rest of our life.

It is sad that in the 2020's some people are disrespectful towards others regarding hygiene. You can see that when many people sneeze, they do not use tissues. Instead, they spit on the ground, drop rubbish anywhere. If adults behave like that, how can they educate children at home to practice proper hygiene?

My grandmother and my parents, as many others, continued to practice the traditional way of farming and preparing food. During summer and autumn there was very little cooking, food was eaten raw. A lot of food needed to be preserved in its natural state and fermented for a long winter. Nothing was wasted; every bit was appreciated and treated with respect. People wouldn't know how long winter was going to last, and how much food needed to be put away all the way to spring.

It is interesting that people without education knew what to do: how to plan and put a system in place that ensured that food was always available to feed the family regardless of how long winter lasted. I remember times when it would start to snow as early as November, and would snow all the way to May. That was six months of hard cold winter. When I say cold, it was that cold that temperatures dropped well below -20 C. That would delay farm work, and having all the seedlings ready to plant in time for harvest before winter arrives again.

Some food was pickled, some dried and some stored in a fresh state (e.g. carrots, potatoes, cabbage, nuts, seeds and some fruits). During winter we were eating the same food for days. We were happy that there was something on the table. Milk and eggs were reserved only for elders and very young children, because there wasn't enough for everyone. Whatever was put on the table was appreciated, and we thanked our mother and father for the food each time and each day.

My grandmother and mother would make bread by hand in large quantity to save on fire wood. Many times there wasn't any flour to make bread, and we would eat polenta or boiled potatoes instead. We made our own butter, and we used it in very small and limited amounts (just smudged it on bread to get the taste). We didn't know that jam existed until the early 1960's.

These days people need to be educated about portion control to manage eating and balancing the budget. Only fresh and nutritious, and mostly plant-based food, was consumed. Occasionally, we ate poultry, pigs or rabbits. I remember I would not eat rabbit because I thought that it was cruel to kill it because it was so cuddly. I was different from my siblings, and my grandmother would call me "softy".

It wasn't as easy as it is today. Now you sit in the car, go to the shops and choose whatever you want. When I see children complain, and throw food on the floor and in the rubbish bin, my memory goes back to my childhood - how I appreciated every bit of food even if it was one week old bread, dry as a rock, it was food. My grandmother would soak the bread in water to soften it, then she would make French toast or dumplings from it - yummy. Most of the time my grandmother would pour hot milk on the bread to feed us. She was a very resourceful lady. My only regret is that I couldn't spend more time with her to learn from her how to use food and herbs as medicine.

In spring we would look under the fruit trees to find any fruit that was covered by snow, and that survived winter. Back then people intuitively knew how to support the body to stay healthy. For breakfast we never ate bread, we ate sauerkraut (fermented cabbage), polenta, eggs, tea and fresh milk straight from the cow (mind you animals were grass feed in a clean environment without the use of any chemicals).

We ate bread only for lunch, with lot of salads and raw vegetables in summer. In winter, we would eat a cooked meal, such as cabbage, legumes, beans, potatoes, hearty soups, and occasionally smoked pork meat, homemade sausages and boiled or roast chicken. Just image feeding nine people with one roast chicken.

All food would be placed in the middle of the table and divided in between nine people. Of course, all meat was home grown/bred free range and totally organically. For dinner, we always had a light meal, such as home-made compote, sour milk (kefir), or home-made fresh cheese (cottage cheese). Food was appreciated and respected. It was consumed in small amounts, easy for the body to digest and use as nutrients and energy. We hardly ever ate biscuits or cakes. Cakes were made only for Easter and Christmas.

I remember it well in spring and autumn after it rained overnight, as children we would disappear in the forest looking for mushrooms. Sometimes we would find big brown field mushrooms as big as a dinner plate. When we stumbled on yellow Chanterelles that was the excitement of the day. These mushrooms have a delicate, beautiful aroma, which when cooked would fill the whole house with their aroma. We were little heroes of the day when we found these. However, this didn't last long as duties on the farm were calling us; there were always jobs waiting to be done.

The water that we drank came from underground, full of essential minerals and micro-minerals that the body needs for growth and development, especially for children. I can see and understand it now, how the problems in eating habits and choice of foods started, and how those poor choices started to affect people's health. Now many times people buy things that are unhealthy for them, and unnecessary. Too many choices can cause people to over eat unhealthy food that creates lots of health problems. The more creative we are with preparing food, the more it can be over processed, and the nutrition in the food can be destroyed.

Personally, I can see how my health changed. As a young child and until the age of 17, I was always healthy living on the land; always eating organic real food, rich in nutrients without any preservatives or processing. Because we ate nutritious food, there was no need for supplements. We only drank water that emerged from under the ground, pure and full of nutrients and essential minerals. We needed to collect the water from the hills with buckets, about a half an hour walk each way. The environment was clean: free of pollution, herbicides and pesticides.

Living in the high country, we didn't have access to seafood. I remember my grandmother chasing us to take liquid fish oil. It smelt so bad that we would hide anywhere we could.   My grandmother would always find us. She was very resourceful; she knew that the mention of food as a reward would bring us out of hiding.   As children, we were so naïve that we always believed what adults told us.

There wasn't any TV or newspapers to educate us; or to distract us. Many of the villagers were unable to read or write. I was living in a village where we didn't have water or toilets in the house. We would go out about 100 meters or more from the house, where we had an outdoor toilet to keep the smell and flies away from the house.

We were living a very simple, healthy life.   Children were learning life values, without the distractions of television, technology and media. We would always eat our meals at the table, listening to adult conversations without interruption. We would speak only when we were asked to.

Today children, even some adults, take health for granted and ignore good health advice. Especially how an unhealthy lifestyle can affect health.   If the family has poor eating habits, consumes alcohol, smokes, uses illegal substances, these are really big issues that can rob a body from nutrition, and change health at a cellular level. In addition, mental health issues can be developed which can disrupt families and lives.

The media, glossy fashion magazines, and food manufacturers are mostly responsible for many teens developing eating disorders, and contributing to their emotional and mental confusion. Young teenagers tend to look at models and celebrities as someone that they want to model. As we know, models in the fashion industry and celebrities are not the best examples to follow.

Times have changed. Parents are busier, work longer hours to make money to support the family, pay school fees, the mortgage and so on. Parents have less time to spend with their children, especially since technology has taken over precious time. Some families are finding it difficult to communicate with each other, and to see early signs of behavior problems.

So many times we see family members sitting at the dinner table focused on technology, instead of using that time to communicate with each other. Once you lose that time, you never get it back. With that is gone an opportunity and possibility to express interest in our children's lives, share wisdom with them, give them a chance to express their feelings, or simply to ask how their day was. These can help children to feel important.

Slowly society started to change, and there was very little practice of the so-called Paleo diet or hunter & gatherer diet. The hunter gatherer diet was around over 12,000 years ago. It involved hunting for animals, fishing and foraging for wild vegetation, honey, etc. for food. Rather than relying on agriculture and growing their own food and farming animals, people would move around to find and hunt for food.

The pure hunter & gatherer diet has changed, and it is impossible to follow it because of changes in farming of different grains and root vegetables. In addition, farming of pigs, cows and poultry replaced hunting for buffalo, deer, rabbit and other game.

I have difficulty understanding how people promote the so called "Paleo diet" in the 2020's. How is that possible? From where do they source the produce?   How is it ethical to promote something that is not possible to follow? We need to educate ourselves to avoid believing everything that we hear and read. The media can be very damaging for our health. We need to understand that as civilization has changed, with that also our quality of life has changed.

Chapter 3
How City Life Changed My Health

As I moved to the city from the country at age 17, it was very exciting. I was given that amazing opportunity to educate myself, and to make something for myself. I remember that day so well. My mother dropped me off to boarding school in Ljubljana (in Slovenia), and I was left there to find my way without knowing anyone.

It was a big step for a country girl to fit into city life, and to be respected as one of the city girls. I also learned to live and to accept city life in a different community, culture and food choices. I even needed to learn to communicate in a different language. It was very difficult, because I was judged and discriminated by how I dressed, and by my hair style. I needed to overcome a lot to fit in.

I noticed changes in the food and water quality, pollution in the city from cars and the environment. People were smoking everywhere; I was exposed to second hand smoking at work and everywhere in that society. Just to go to the coffee shop for lunch, there was a cloud of smoke sitting above your head. The majority of people were smoking.

In less than a year, my health started to be affected. My immune system became so weak that I was constantly sick compared to my life before I came to the city. Not only in winter, but in summer too. In the hottest time of summer (August in Europe), I would get such a bad flu that my GP couldn't work out what was going on. I was constantly on antibiotics.

When I look back at what was going on, it is no wonder why I was getting sick! The city water was missing vital nutrients, chemical substances were added to the water that my body was reacting to. Food was high in sugar, animal fats, simple carbohydrates and additives, and highly processed. Life was very different in the city from that in the high country.

In the city, a lot of fatty food and cakes were consumed, as well as alcohol and smoking. People were indulging themselves in bad habits. Instead of water, soft drinks were in fashion, especially for the wealthy. You could see a different attitude in them. Those less fortunate were judged by how they dressed. In restaurants, even waitresses were giving judgmental looks to people who couldn't afford to indulge themselves like the wealthy ones. The more food you ordered, the more respected you were.

I needed to grow up very fast to fit into that unhealthy society. At the same time, it was important for me to start to develop new friends. I went out to the cinema with them, and then we treated ourselves with cake and coffee. I do understand now how important it is to have a good 8-9 hours of sleep every night for the body to rejuvenate itself. At that time I would have 5-6 hours of sleep on most occasions. Because I was working shift work in the hospitality industry, every day I was exposed to second hand smoking, and was consuming unhealthy, unbalanced and undernourished food. I am very proud of myself that I never indulged in consuming alcohol or smoking.

Now we can see how we are affected by bad food choices, chemicals and preservatives that we consume. Even when we want to make healthy choices, it it very hard because manufacturers are not clearly listing ingredients on packaging so that consumers can make educated choices. Many personal care products are as bad because they contain petrochemicals and carcinogens, which mimic hormones that are potentially dangerous for humans.

Mimic hormones are synthetic estrogens that our immune system recognizes as harmless, until they are absorbed into our system. Once they are in the system, the immune system starts to react. In addition, there is environmental poisoning that is added to crops and drinking water, our cleaning products are full of harmful chemicals, and pollution is in the air. These harmful substances are found everywhere, and affect our health.

I asked myself how so many babies and young children are diagnosed with life threatening illnesses. Children as young as one year old are diagnosed with allergies and respiratory problems. I never heard about such illnesses while I was living in the high country up to 1960's. In the country we didn't have doctors and, as children, we were never immunized until the late 1950's.

Once the modern world started to take over, smoking became fashionable, over consumption of alcohol and modern food, fancy and highly processed cakes, and pre-packaged fast food all started to become part of the good life. Was it really the good life or poisoning our body to destroy our immune defenses, and set us up for so many health problems later in life?

Now I understand why my health was so sensitive - because the vital nutrients to support good health were missing from my every day eating plan. My stress levels were extremely high, working shift work and looking after the family, and all the other duties that we needed to do as women and mothers. There were no support groups that women and mothers could go to for help or to just simply talk about problems in life. If you did confide in people around you, they would make fun of you and see you as a weak person unable to manage your life and look after your family. So it was better to keep it to yourself, and to do the best that you could.

My health problems didn't stop there, and followed me to Australia. Because of unhealthy eating and an over use of antibiotics over a number of years, I developed poor digestion and an out of balance yeast infection, Candida Ambilica. I lived with it for over 30 years before I started to understand how to deal with it.

Up to the late 1990's doctors were using antibiotics as a treatment for this condition which created more problems for intestinal flora, and destroyed the good gut bacteria. Because doctors did not know how to diagnose and treat Candida, every couple of years I needed to remove uterine cysts. To make matters worse, in my early 40's my GP put me on (HRT) synthetic hormone replacement therapy. He also insisted that I needed to stay on HRT regardless of my concerns about it.

After staying on HRT for over 9 years, I started to experience more health problems. That was very difficult to understand, because at that time I was always very conscious of healthy living and looking after my family so that they stay healthy. Working in the hospitality industry for over 35 years, the high stress and shift work started to have an effect on me and my health. I was overworked; my body started to show signs of exhaustion and stress. I knew that I needed to make changes to be able to look after my family and myself.

I decided to sell my restaurant (after running it for 10 years), and to take a break. I took my first holiday after working for 28 years. I took 3 months off to travel through Europe. On my return flight back, I decided to change my career. I was done with shift work and stressful work in hospitality. It was a difficult decision because I didn't know what I wanted to change to.

I went back to working in hospitality for another two years. During that time, I had two work injuries to my neck and shoulders, due to heavy lifting. After the second injury, I was off work for four years. Over that time I was going from specialist to specialist, popping painkillers like lollies, until I asked myself what I am doing to my health.

I was pretending that I was happy; people who knew me well could see that something was going on with me, especially my daughter Vesna. She encouraged me to start to look for options. She knew that I needed to start working again. The only problem was to find a job that I could manage with my injuries. As soon as my previous injuries were mentioned in jobs that I applied for, my chances of getting the job were ruined. The only option that I could see was to start something completely new, something that would give me the flexibility to work without causing more pain to myself.

Chapter 4
Changing Career in My Late 50's

An old saying says "it is never too late to start something new". I was in my 50's, and when most people think of planning for retirement, I started to think of changing my career. Now I am very proud that I did, and what I have achieved. The changes I made gave me an education and knowledge as to how to live a healthier life. I was desperate to get out of an unhealthy situation. Because I was working without a break from the age of 17 until age 45, I was stressed about being able to find a job that I could do after the injuries.

I decided to do something different: something that would help me change my life and to improve my health, and to be able to help and educate others. For almost one year, I was searching and attending different health seminars. In the process and after working with food for over 35 years, I found there is a big gap to be filled - to really understand healthy living, the obstacles that we face every day in a society with unhealthy choices of food, and a polluted environment.

First, I completed Reiki (energy healing) level 1 and level 2, followed by the Master level. That helped me to help myself, to learn how to relax, and to be more focused on positive outcomes. It wasn't something that I could do for a living at that time, because I was searching for something that I was really passionate about. So I continued my search. I completed a Diploma in Food and Environmental Allergies as I felt it is very close to my past education, and my passion for working with food.

As part of my Diploma, I was working with my case study client for my final exam: a client who suffered from severe eczema for over 18 years. I was able to help my client to overcome eczema. More importantly, my client has been continuously free from eczema for well over 22 years now. I educated my client how to implement healthy eating, how to avoid chemicals in the home and in personal care products, so as to avoid recreating ill health again. I realized that I needed more education in nutrition to be able to help people and myself to achieve best results, and to change ill people's lives.

Completing the Diploma in Clinical Nutrition allowed me to understand how the body systems work together, and what is needed to bring the body back into balance. I was able to help myself to stop taking HRT, and to supplement my body with more natural herbal supplements that didn't cause side effects as synthetic HRT did. (Please ask your medical/health professional to help you to make any changes you wish). I was able to reduce my body weight by 20 kilos in the first year. That alone helped me to identify and to ask for help to address the emotional issues that I was experiencing from childhood.

I started to search how I could do that without medication. My search led me to a highly educated Neuro Linguistic Programming (NLP) and Hypnotherapy Master Practitioner. I really enjoyed working with her, and I was impressed by the excellent results she achieved with me in a very short period of time. I was so inspired by her professionalism that I decided to become a Master Practitioner in the field, and to help people with emotional issues. Now I can help people with different needs, help them to change their life style and to choose healthier habits and behaviors.

My education in the food industry was very helpful when it came to creating healthy recipes, and planning healthy eating plans. I am happy now that I gained the education to be able to help individuals with a wider range of issues. Yet again, I was helping everyone around me, and neglected to look after myself. I realised that in helping others I needed to be healthy, to reward myself for the hard work, and to learn to take time out for myself.

In 2001 I decided that it was time to have a family reunion in Croatia, because all of my siblings were living in different continents. It was over 38 years since we were all together as a family. In July 2001 we all surprised our parents; it was the day that they were waiting for. We had the time of our life at the home where we were all born and grew up. A lot of memories and laughter. We were so loud that passers-by joined us in celebrating our family reunion. This was my third time back home. I was happy, and it was a great reward to myself for my hard work, and my study achievements. Sadly, both my parents passed away 10 months later. It seemed like they were waiting for that family reunion to see us all together for the last time.

Chapter 5
Recognizing Warning Signs & Diagnosis

In our busy everyday life, it can be difficult to recognize what is happening inside our body. So many things are happening that we can ignore the day after day discomfort. The longer we ignore this, the worse it gets. When we are in tune with our inner self, and pay attention to the discomfort and even the smallest changes, we can prevent our health from deteriorating to the level where we lose control of it.

I started to notice many warning signs at the same time that made it more difficult to work out what could be happening to my internal health. These warning signs included:
- My body pH was dropping (my body had become acidic)
- My Vitamin D levels were dropping
- My body inflammation was rising (ESR levels)
- The candida (yeast overgrowth) was constantly present
- My digestion was suffering
- I had daily bloating and cramps
- Blood spotting started

At the time when I noticed that my body pH dropped to just under 4.5 pH (very low), I started to worry because it was a big drop from 7.365 pH (which is normal). I started to look at any possible causes. Initially, it was difficult to pin point what caused the body to be out of balance to that extent. My body was out of balance because a number of different elements and symptoms were present.

As we now know, vitamin D is important to protect us from many different cancers, and to support the body's bone structure and other body systems. My level of vitamin D dropped to 20 despite me already taking 2000 ui per day of vitamin D3 supplements. I expressed my concern to my specialist; he ran a number of tests and he couldn't find anything that I needed to worry about. His reply was that my body does not need a high level of vitamin D. I wasn't happy because I knew that the normal level for vitamin D should be at least 70. I thought there must be a better explanation, and started to do my own research.

The Inflammation level in my blood test (ESR) showed 37, which is way too high. My CRP level (which measures infections in the body) was above 10, again too high. A safe ESR level is under 20, and a safe CRP level is under 4.

I know that when the body starts to become too acidic, all the internal body systems are under enormous stress. I also know that changes must be made in nutrition, including an alkaline eating plan, to help the body to eliminate acid and to bring it back into balance.

To deal with each of the above issues, I needed to make big changes in my life style. I changed my eating plan to be totally alkaline, and organic for 3 months. After all this planning and effort, little had changed. I was disappointed, and was looking for answers. I needed to find the root cause of the problem. I also knew that something bigger was happening in my body, and that I needed to find answers very fast.

At the time, I had a really bad gut feeling. At the same time, I was telling myself it cannot be, it is not possible that it is cancer. If it is, where in the body is it? I was comforting myself with the knowledge that there is no family history of cancer. I started to put the pieces together by looking at my health history all the way back in time when I started to live in the city. As I started to record my past health history, I started to get the bigger picture of what was happening. I needed to narrow this down before I saw my GP.

In early 2009, I started to experience some symptoms that I couldn't understand so I looked for answers. By the time I put the missing pieces together, it was all too late. I was diagnosed with gynecological cancer in August 2010. I was lucky to have the education and knowledge to recognize at an early stage that something is not right with me. I followed my instinct to investigate, and to do the tests to get answers. I was very lucky that my (female) GP took the time to hear me out, worked together with me to find out what was going on in time, and took the appropriate action towards it.

To have a medical doctor at your side that is willing to listen, and to take the time to explain things to you is very important. Because I was very confused, it felt as if my brain was on fire. A lot of different emotions were going on, and many questions in my head that I didn't know the answers to.

I started to feel disappointed in myself – why was I not able to take better care of myself? My emotions were taking over my clear thinking; I could not sleep. I was lying in bed, and all sort of things were going through my head, so many what ifs? When it was time to get up, I was so exhausted. My entire day continued to be full of worries, I could not think. I decided to ask for help, and to address what was going on in my head. Once I addressed the emotional issues, I was able to take control of what I needed to do and to ask for appropriate help and advice. Again, Dr. Vesna was there to help me with the emotional issues.

Never in my wildest dreams did it cross my mind that I would be in a situation where my life could be in that kind of danger. At the time, it was even more difficult for me to accept the diagnosis because I never consumed alcohol, never smoked (although I had been exposed to second hand smoke) or lived a wild unhealthy life. I became a statistic as a cancer patient.

In my life, I overcame so many obstacles and difficulties, and I always had the courage and energy to deal with. This was different. I knew that it was there, yet I couldn't see it, touch it or feel it. I can honestly say that was the most difficult time of my life.

The day of the diagnosis, and the following two days, I felt as if I was having a bad dream. I kept saying to myself that it cannot be happening to me. Then reality kicked in. I received a call from the hospital to confirm my appointment with the oncologist. My mind was working a thousand miles per second. I kept a positive face, yet inside I was miles away looking for the answers. I felt as if I was locked in a cage, no way out; emotionally and mentally I was trapped.

I started to think of my daughter, how badly she would take the news. I needed to be strong for her, to show her how to stay positive and that together we will come through this in good health. I could see that she was very stressed. Through my mind went question after question: what do I need to do to reassure her that I am going pull through this? I decided to include her on this journey so that we could support each other.

I asked her to keep me positive. I am so grateful to have such a caring and supportive daughter.

I am grateful to my GP for listening to my concerns, and acting fast because time was of the essence. It was important to get all the tests done in the shortest time possible, and to get me to the gynecologist/oncologist on time. When I saw the oncologist, I did not even have a chance to sit down in her office, and without any preparation she told me abruptly "Bad news, it is cancer." She then sent me to a specialist oncologist in a different section of the hospital. It was a shock mentally and emotionally to hear such news.

When I saw the oncologist, all I could hear him say is that I needed to have a full hysterectomy to avoid cancer returning. When I asked him why I needed to remove the ovaries, his reply was, "you won't need them because you are over 60." At the time, I was so confused and in emotional and mental shock that my brain stopped working. If only the oncologist was as understanding as my GP, it would have been easier emotionally and mentally. I agreed to proceed with the surgery, which I regret to this day. I should have asked for some time to get my thoughts together or for a second opinion.

On the day of the surgery while lying on the preparation table, very drowsy having already been administered a general anesthetic, the specialist surgeon whispered in my ear that they will do some radiotherapy too. Luckily, I was aware enough to respond, and asked him to only do the surgery I authorized them in the paperwork I had signed earlier that morning. This is the last thing that I remember until I was brought into the recovery room after surgery.

It was an 8-hour surgery, and my body was suspended upside down the whole time. After surgery while lying in my hospital room, I remember the nurse placing a morphine pump in my left hand, and telling me to press that button when I feel pain. As soon as I heard that, I dropped the pump out of my hand. I did not want any morphine because it is highly addictive. The next morning when the nurse came to check on me, the first thing she said was that I did not use any morphine. I replied that I did not need it, and she told me that I must be in pain because I just had major surgery. She walked away.

Every half an hour, different nurses came to check on me and offered me pain killers. I refused each time. Little did they know that I had my pain under control naturally, using self-hypnosis. In the meantime, the woman in the bed next to me was in agony after having the same surgery as I did. She was screaming in pain the whole night, and pumping morphine the whole time.

The only medication I was on was for an underactive thyroid. On the second day after surgery, I asked the nurse for my thyroid medication. The nurse brought me the wrong tablet. I noticed the tablet was the wrong shape, and told her that it was not my medication. After that I lost trust in the hospital. When the surgeon came to see me for a routine checkup, I asked him if I could go home. He questioned whether I was ready to go home, I replied I was ready to go home. He examined me first, then he told me that he never saw anyone who healed so fast after a major surgery. He agreed that I could go home.

My check-up for 6 weeks' time was booked and I was released from hospital. I was released without any instructions or information as to how to access a support group if I needed any emotional support. Three days later, a letter arrived from a cancer association asking for donations, without any concern for how I am feeling or how my family is coping. It is beyond me why they treat patients differently.

From my experience, breast cancer patients get so much support and care, while patients with gynecological cancer get so little support. After so many women lose the battle with gynecological cancer, you would think that all patients regardless of the type of cancer or what part of body is affected by cancer, a program would be in place to give support to each person as soon as possible to avoid unnecessary stress for the patient and their family members. I hope things have improved for the better since 2010.

Ten years on, I was still hearing the specialist's words, "it is bad news, it is cancer." I was working very hard to stay positive, in control and to avoid getting stressed. Each time when I went for the check up, those words were buzzing around my mind like an annoying fly that wouldn't go away.

Now I know how cancer patients feel - hopeless when they are diagnosed with cancer, especially if they are emotionally and mentally vulnerable. The rest of the family becomes hopeless because they find it difficult to support the patient. We mean well when we start to feel sorry for ill people. Believe me, it makes it worse.

I made a decision as soon I started to have the initial tests, that feeling sorry for myself and others feeling sorry for me will make the situation even worse. For that reason, I made the decision to only share my health challenges with family and a few friends. I asked them to support me, and to keep me positive and free from stress. The last thing that I wanted was for anyone to feel sorry for me, and to keep me in a negative state.

One thing that I have learned during my NLP and Hypnotherapy studies is that our conscious and unconscious mind need to support each other, and that staying positive will make me stronger to deal with any situation. I believe now that this is very important for every person that is affected by an illness, and their family too. Together, they need to be able to support each other, and look towards successful recovery and healing.

Family members also need to give space to the ill person, and respect what they want. They need to avoid constantly making decisions for them, and ignoring what the ill person wants. The ill person is under enormous stress already, and putting extra stress on them can easily push them into depression.

It is wonderful to have visitors. I only had ones who were positive, and I kept the visits short to avoid extra stress. Family members also need to look after their own emotional and mental health, and to ask for help to avoid getting stressed. It is important to ask for professional help if you feel that you need it. Addressing any emotional issues will allow you to think clearly, to make better decisions, and to stay positive and focused on your healing journey.

Chapter 6
My Plan for Support and Healing

Now that I had the surgery and I just recovered from the mental shock, reality started to kick in about what to do next. I had great advice from Dr. Vesna to do what is right for me. As this is my journey of recovery, only I need to be happy with what I do next in my life. She suggested to take pen and paper, and to start making a plan of what I wanted.

Planning my healing journey helped me to avoid stress and focusing on illness. Instead, I focused on the future, how I can be healthy again, and rejuvenate my body for optimal health. So I did. Most of the time I spent in my back yard. It was peaceful, relaxing and self-empowering. I felt that I was in charge, and I decided my recovery and treatment:

1. I decided to share my healing journey only with close family members, and with my closest friends. I could rely on them to be there for me, and that they would support me. I wanted to avoid the extra stress of dealing with negative people; I didn't have the time or the energy for negativity. I asked all of them to be positive around me, and to keep me positive too.

2. I decided to avoid making any decisions before I had the time to re-evaluate them, and to see what options I have. A second opinion is very helpful.

3. Most importantly, I asked my family and friends to respect my decisions, and to give me space where I can relax and have time for myself.

4. I always had my daughter, Vesna, with me for emotional and mental support when I went for check-ups to the hospital.

5. I planned my eating plan, exercise and supplementation where necessary. Once I put that plan in place; I started to plan how to communicate with the medical team, and get them on my side to understand what is important to me. It was challenging because the oncologist wasn't very happy with my decisions. I asked him to let me take my time to go step by step with my decisions because it was too much to deal with all at the same time.

I took it day by day for the first year of recovery. After the first year when I received the all clear from the oncologist, I was able to make long term plans. I felt that I needed to share my story and my journey with others so they have at least some knowledge about taking good care of their own health.

The most important question that I asked myself was "how will I deal with the oncologist and the medical team?" I wanted to stay in control, and to make educated decisions that were best for me. Of course, I took on board what the oncologist had in mind, and I incorporated that into my plan so I could get the best outcome. I planned the questions that I was going to ask, and I was persistent to get the answers. Because I did not get answers to all my questions pre surgery, I could have made a different decision, and could have had a different outcome. I learned that I needed to get the answer with which I am happy during my pre-surgery consultation. That was my biggest learning.

I started to plan my healing journey. I researched nutrition books written by experts in the field. I combined this research with all my prior knowledge, and made a plan from the start. I changed my eating plan, my environment, my water, and my mindset. It was important to create time, and a quiet place for me where I can relax and have space from being over-crowded. One thing that I needed to be clear about was to avoid having too many visitors at the same time because I needed time to re-energize my body, physically and emotionally. I asked visitors to come when it was the best time for me.

I knew that I needed to do whatever was necessary to stay positive and strong; to learn that it is ok to ask for help, to rest as much as I needed, to eat healthy natural fresh food, drink clean water and sleep as much as I needed. Only then would I be able to take control of my health, and my life again. I was and am very lucky to have a supportive daughter that is continuously there for me, and willing to help and respect my wishes and decisions. Most important for me was staying one step ahead, looking after myself and making the decisions that are right for me.

Looking back on all that had happened, I know that everything happened for a reason. I have learned that by not following my instinct, looking after everyone else first and leaving myself last, brought me to where I was with my health. Now my priorities are to look after myself first. Because if I am healthy, I'm able to look after my family and everyone else whom may need my help.

I am very disappointed because I didn't get any advice from the medical team in hospital about nutrition life changes, or emotional and mental health, or support for my family to cope during this journey. Nor was any information given to me as to how and where to get help if I needed it. I was lucky that I knew that I needed to ask for help. How many patients are less fortunate, and they do not know that asking for help can make a big difference to their recovery.

I believe that regardless of whether you are a private or public patient, we all deserve to get the equal and best advice and treatment that is available. I can see that much more needs to be done to help less fortunate people have the education and support in difficult times. It would be even better to educate the community about how to prevent illnesses in the first place.

From my life experience, I wonder what a wonderful life people would have if young parents were presented with life strategies so that they could educate and protect their children from a very young age to live healthy stress-free lives, free from bullying and bad influences. As God is my witness, I had plenty of emotional, mental and physical bullying since childhood until I was almost 40 years old. I did my best to deal with this. All I could do on many occasions was to suppress all my emotions and problems, hoping they would go away. I know now that was wishful thinking, they didn't go away. Suppressing emotions created more health problems.

We do the best that we can, and make the best choices we can in life. It is important that we learn from negative experiences, and create positive environments. Then we can use that experience and learning to help educate and support others with information on how and where help is available when they need it.

Chapter 7
How I Dealt with Life Challenging Decisions

I was determined to overcome my health challenge, and to learn the lesson I needed to learn. I asked myself many questions, the most important ones were:

- Where did it all go wrong?
- Why me?
- How can I fix it?
- What do I need to learn from it?
- How do I avoid making the same mistakes in the future?

Once I was able to answer all of the above questions, I gave myself permission to start my healing journey. I knew that I needed to be prepared for challenges. I always had plan B to fall back on to avoid being disappointed, and, most importantly, to avoid giving up. I was always moving forward regardless of how challenging it was. One step at a time was the key.

- I dealt with my emotional and mental health to ensure that I was ready to deal with whatever the future presented to me. I cleaned up my past from traumas and emotional blockages. Then I made sure that I was physically ready, and allowed my body to rest and regain strength that it needed to start the healing process.

- I planned and created a healthy eating plan for me to nourish my body, and to strengthen my immune system.

- I found and implemented appropriate supplements to support my immune system, and incorporated daily exercise that was right for me.

- I wanted my family to stay healthy so I started to prepare food that they can eat to stay healthy at the same time. This made it less obvious that I was on a special eating plan, and prevented the constant reminder that I was the one that needed special attention.

- Most importantly, I needed to remind myself daily to stay on track, to avoid overdoing it, and to prevent stressing myself mentally or physically. I made sure I took time out for me, and had plenty of uninterrupted sleep at night.

The biggest issue for me was dealing with my emotions. I was brought up to be strong, and that showing emotions makes a person weak. So I learned to suppress my emotions to be able to deal with a hard life, the bullying and a male dominated era. Now I know that suppressing emotions is toxic and poison for our soul, body and mind. It was a lot to take on emotionally, mentally and physically. I created a mental plan to take each day one at a time, and to take baby steps forward.

I dealt with the surgery and the pathology tests first. Then I needed to wait to see the oncologist for the results. First, I felt as though I was in a pressure cooker ready to explode. Not knowing what the next visit to the oncologist would present me with.

The first visit, 6 weeks after surgery, was the most nerve wrecking. My daughter noticed this, and asked the oncologist if it is appropriate for me to go away on a 4-hour driving trip and a weekend away. He agreed as long I avoided any heavy lifting. My daughter took me to Bright, amongst beautiful scenery and a peaceful clean environment. I felt a range of emotions that I never experienced before.

My daughter, Vesna, worked very hard to keep me busy. She helped to keep my mind on the beautiful scenery and surroundings, and to enjoy the peaceful environment and wild life around us. I did my best; I didn't want to disappoint her because she put so much time and effort to make me happy and comfortable. I remember that walk along the river on an early rainy morning with my daughter, seeing young rabbits hiding under the bushes, ducks swimming in the river - it was so peaceful, and just the right remedy that I needed at the time.

I needed to learn to accept the loss of my feminine organs. I felt I needed to allow myself grieving time, while also learning to nourish my body's endocrine system to function without the missing organs. It is very important for their healing to recovery, that women allow themselves to grieve and accept the loss of the feminine organs.

I needed to stay as positive and as calm as possible. Because if you start to panic and lose control, you could develop anxiety and depression. At my first visit to the oncologist after the operation, I did not get much explanation only that my body is healing well. Then I needed to wait another 3 months for the next round of tests and results, hoping that they will be all clear from cancer. I did anything I could to keep myself busy to avoid thinking about this.

When the time finally arrived to see the oncologist for the test results, those 20 minutes of waiting in the waiting room became the longest 20 minutes of my life. When the oncologist said that everything is healing nicely and that the tests are all clear, free of cancer, that was the best news that I received in a long time. It felt like a truck fell off my shoulders, and I was able to breathe and think again. Now I needed to take it easy, and to have a check-up every three months for the first year. I was ok with that. It took a lot of my energy to go through all the tests and examinations. I felt as though I was never at home. Between August 2010 and January 2011, I visited the hospital for tests and oncologist appointments 21 times.

I was very upfront with the oncologist - I wanted to be a part of all decisions and choice of treatment, before and after an operation. He suggested Radiotherapy after the operation. I decided to take one step at a time, and asked to have the operation first, and then to take the next step as appropriate. Because the cancer was at an early stage and it hadn't spread, I decided to not have radiotherapy. Instead, I focused on how I can make changes to help my body to heal, and to strengthen my immune system to support my body.

Honestly, I was very surprised with the oncologist's attitude. Let's just say that he didn't support my decision; he was so in my face that my daughter needed to ask him to stop making me more stressed. My GP continued to be very supportive, and ran the necessary tests to help me to be more relaxed, and to have peace of mind. It is very important to have your GP on your side. 3rd November 2011 was one year after the surgery. I was so relived that my healing and recovery was going from strength to strength.

That was a big step forward. Now I needed to get back into what we call a normal life. There is no such thing because every discomfort or pain brings back that memory, questions, and what ifs. Once the organs have been removed out of your body, you feel that emptiness, and that the body is missing those organs. Personally, I am feeling it every day.

Now another problem presented itself. I started to put on weight, regardless of walking every day and how well I looked after my eating. Just imagine you drive your car to the mechanic, and he does not put all the parts back. You will notice very quickly that your car is driving differently, and sooner or later your car will feel the effects of the missing parts. That is what happens to our body when the organs have been removed, it is never the same. Yes, we continue our life as normal as we can, hoping for the best.

It is important to be realistic. We hear many stories and read many books that were written by celebrities, and how they went through their cancer recovery journey. As I already mentioned, we are all unique and individual. Our body reacts differently to emotions and the environment, and celebrities are in a different financial position to many people. Many of them can employ personal chefs, housekeepers, gardeners, fitness trainers, personal doctors to visit them at home, baby sitters and other help and support. How many individuals can afford to create this life style to support their healing process? I know many individuals who have difficulties going through treatments, and have a hard time to manage life. So be realistic, and avoid focusing on celebrity lifestyles, and how they survive cancer treatments.

Instead, I focused on my unique situation, and how I can create the healing process for me to get the best outcome possible. I am just an ordinary person like thousands of other women, needing to work hard to earn a living and to pay the bills. I can relate to you in everyday situations better than any celebrities out there.

My suggestion to all women and men who are going through cancer or any other illness is to find a supportive, positive friend or support group. This will assist you to support each other, share your concerns, lend each other an ear, and laugh together. In our busy everyday life, we can forget to laugh. As the saying goes: "laughter is the best medicine". How very true. While we laugh, we are unable to have negative thoughts and think about our problems.

Some doctors have a different theory that once women reach over 60 years of age, they can live without their feminine organs. Yes, we can live without our feminine organs; the question is how well can we live without them? Only women who have been through an experience of illness can feel it, and understand other women.

Because it is our body, each woman understands her body better than anyone else. We need to go through a healing process, and understand that we are still the same person that we were before any illness. Only now we are stronger, and able to share and support others who are going through similar health challenges.

A woman's body is very complex when it comes to reproductive organs. When they have been removed, our body goes out of balance. All hormones are out of balance. Our health is dependent on hormones. If reproductive organs are missing, insufficient hormones are produced, putting all bodily systems out of balance. Educate yourself and ask your GP for options because synthetic hormones may not be the best option for everyone, especially if you have a family history of cancer. The appendix at the back of this book contains resources to assist you.

As I mentioned, our reproductive system is very important for our health. Estrogen and Progesterone play important roles in supporting bone density to prevent Osteoporosis. Ask your doctor for advice to help you support bone density.

Also ask your GP about herbal support or for Bio-Indentical Hormone Replacement therapy. Look for information to educate yourself before you go to the GP. This will help you to have an informed conversation with your GP, and make an informed decision that is right for you. A great book with lots of information for women is written by Jonathan V. Wright, MD and Lane Lenard, PhD called "Stay Young & Sexy with Bio-Identical Hormone Replacement".

Chapter 8
Life is Full of Surprises

You would think that one year since the cancer had been surgically removed and all is clear, that you would be more aware of what is going on with your body. Despite doing everything possible to stay healthy, I started to have uneasy feelings around my abdomen, almost a nagging pain, and yet I wasn't able to pin point what was going on. I again expressed my concern to my GP. By now, we had established a good relationship as a patient and doctor. I knew that I could trust her to do what is right for me. Blood tests showed that the liver was not showing any abnormality. Yet, I was not convinced.

I started to have a strange feeling that something is going on, that I needed to look deeper to find the root cause of the problem. I asked how could we be certain that there is no problem with the liver. To give me peace of mind, my GP ordered an ultrasound of the liver. Surprise, surprise, the ultrasound test came back as "fatty liver". We were both puzzled. Because I had been very conscious of my food selection, how is that possible?

The next question was how do we deal with it. My GP said: There is no medication for this, and there is not much I can do about it if you are on a healthy eating plan already. I would not accept this. I was determined to get an answer to my question, and so I started to do research through all my nutrition books. First, I identified that there are two types of fatty liver: "alcoholic and non-alcoholic fatty liver syndrome". I was already closer to the answer because I never consumed alcohol. I continued to research how to deal with "non-alcoholic fatty liver". As the name says, there is a difference between alcoholic and non-alcoholic fatty liver.

Now remember that most illness takes time to develop, often over a number of years. Non-alcoholic fatty liver affects people who consume a lot of sugary foods such as: any products made from white flour, highly processed foods with added sugars, cakes, soft drinks/energy drinks, and taking medication long-term. Now it all started to make sense to me. Fatty liver does not happen over the short term, it is an accumulation process of stress and lifestyle on the liver.

The liver is a very important organ; it performs over 500 jobs every day. When it becomes overloaded with toxic matter and fat day after day, it starts to get sluggish. Bread, pasta, sugars and processed foods, fried food, animal proteins, lard, margarines, butter, pre-packaged food, even sugar from too much fresh fruit, are converted into fat. In turn, that overloaded fat ends up in the liver.

As I continued my research, I found a good explanation and very good information on a group of Melbourne doctors' website www.digestivehealth.com.au. I combined that information with what I found during my search in my nutrition books. I put a plan in place. I changed my eating plan again to eat a lot more green-leafed vegetables, and cut down to 2 pieces of fruit per day. Previously, I was eating a lot of fruit to get extra nutritional value and anti-oxidants.

During this search, I discovered that eating large amounts of fruit can put the liver under stress, as it processes the extra sugars (fructose). Also, there is the possibility of developing type 2 diabetes. I drank 2-3 liters of alkaline water a day to help flush out the fat and the toxins. I started the day with half a fresh lemon, juiced in 200 ml. of warm alkaline water. I also walked every day, first thing in the morning. I will share my full plan with you in next two chapters.

Chapter 9
How Sugars and Fats Affect Our Liver and Our Health

Yes, some of us like more sugary and sweet foods than others. Occasionally, and in very small amounts, it is OK to consume these if you are a reasonably healthy person, and I really mean HEALTHY.

Are you someone who needs sugar hits for energy? Do you have a habit of snacking on sweet food, going for energy drinks, the biscuit box, or chocolates? When you are feeling stressed or emotional, are you running a pattern of emotional eating where you are constantly going to the fridge or the pantry to suppress your emotions?

Sugar is very addictive. If you attempt to simply avoid it, you can start to experience withdrawal symptoms such as: headaches, sleeping problems, irritability, become angry, etc. All of these can lead to more health issues. There is also the possibility of creating addictions to food, alcohol, or other substances, which are definitely bad for you. It is a good idea to ask for professional help to address emotional issues rather than to suppress them with food. Suppressing emotions with food is unhealthy for your body, and especially for your liver. Every time you suppress your emotions, you are creating more health issues and may be supporting deeper habits or addictions.

For example, anger is directly connected to liver health. If you suppress your anger as I did, it can affect your liver. When I learned that I have cancer, I was very angry at myself for not taking better care of myself. It had an effect on my liver, until I dealt with the anger and other emotional issues. Once again, I asked Dr. Vesna to help me to address my emotions and emotional eating, and to create healthier eating habits.

After eating too much fruit or fructose that is added to food, most of the metabolic burden rests on your liver. Take for example dried fruit, it is loaded with fructose. Because all the water is dehydrated out of that fruit, dried fruit is smaller in size than fresh fruit, yet it has more sugar than fresh fruit. Therefore, avoid snacking too much on dried fruit to avoid overloading your system with fructose.

So where does all of this fructose go once you consume it? Our body cannot use fructose directly as energy, and most of the fructose that we consume goes directly to our liver to be converted into glucose. When our liver is overloaded with fructose, it also ramps up fat production which means more lipids in blood. That is bad for our heart. It turns into fat which means more fat deposits throughout your body, especially around the abdomen. That was my problem. I started to grow around the abdomen, and my body weight started to increase. That was a very unpleasant feeling, and I knew that I needed to bring it under control.

Too much fructose can also increase uric acid, and create other health issues such as: raised blood pressure, damage the kidneys, and create inflammation. Chronically inflamed blood vessels lead to heart attacks and strokes. Chronic inflammation can lead to some cancers. Elevated blood sugar levels also lead to weight gain, abdominal obesity, diabetes, increased cholesterol, and non-alcoholic fatty liver disease. It is a vicious circle, and you need to stop it before it gets out of hand.

Sugar can create so many health issues in the body. We need to consume sugar in moderation or even better in very low quantities to keep the body in balance. It is healthier to eat fresh fruit. If you consume dried fruit, have these in very small amounts, limit these to one serving per day. One serving is 2 tablespoons of raisins or 2 to 3 apricot halves or 3 dates or 1 large fig.

There is another downside to dried fruit. They are often sprayed with a sugar solution before drying to make them taste sweeter. Dried cranberries and cherries are notorious for this. Dried bananas are even fried in oil before they are sweetened with added sugars, then go through the drying process. All dried fruit goes through a heating process, and during that process they lose a lot of nutritional value. If you choose to eat dried fruit, it is best to choose organic, sun-dried fruit.

Below is a handy chart to help you to estimate how much fructose you are getting in your daily food. Remember, you are also likely getting additional fructose and other forms of sugars in prepackaged foods, soft drinks, cakes, bread, pasta, etc. since it is hidden in nearly all food.

Instead of simple carbohydrates, always choose healthier complex carbohydrates such as: spelt products, basmati or brown rice, quinoa, lots off fresh food preferably organically and locally grown. Always read the label on packaged food. When you prepare food yourself, you are more in control of what is in your food.

FRUIT	SERVING SIZE	GRAMS - FRUCTOSE
Lime	1 medium	0
Lemon	1 medium	0.6
Cranberries	1 cup	0.7
Passionfruit	1 medium	0.9
Guava	1 medium	1.1
Prune	1 medium	1.2
Apricot	1 medium	1.3
Date	1 medium	2.6
Cantaloupe	1/8 of medium	2.8
Raspberries	1 cup	3.0
Kiwifruit	1 medium	3.4
Blackberries	1 cup	3.5
Star fruit	1 medium	3.6
Sweet Cherries	10 medium	3.8
Strawberries	1 cup	3.8
Sour Cherries	10 medium	4.0
Pineapple	1 medium slice	4.0
Grapefruit, pink	½ medium	4.3
Boysenberries	1 cup	4.6
Tangerine	1 medium	4.8
Mandarin	1 medium	4.8
Nectarine	1 medium	5.4
Peach	1 medium	5.9
Orange	1 medium	6.1
Papaya	½ medium	6.3
Honeydew	1/8 medium	6.7
Banana	1 medium	7.1
Blueberries	1 cup	7.4
Apple, whole	1 medium	9.5
Persimmon	1 medium	10.6
Watermelon	1/16 medium	11.3
Pear	1 medium	11.8
Raisins	¼ cup	12.3

The above chart may help you to count your sugar content when you are shopping. Always go for products that contain under 10 grams of sugar per 100 grams. Always have your shopping list with you, and only buy what is on the list.

Keep in mind that dried fruit contains more fructose than fresh fruit of the same quantity and type.

The other sugars that need to be taken into considerations when we are planning our meal are: dextrose, corn sugar, ethanol, xylitol, glycerol, sorbitol, malitol, erythritol, sucralose, aspartame, saccharin, agave, honey, stevia. During my research, I learned that stevia is healthy, and is almost calorie free. It is very sweet, and you will need it in very small amounts. You can substitute it for sugar when cooking, baking or adding sweetness to any food.

Just recently I discovered monk fruit sweetener. It is a very healthy substitute for sugar, has 0 sugar and is gluten free. If you are consuming more than 20 grams of sugar per day, you need to stop, find out where your sugar intake is coming from, and re-evaluate your eating plan.

My Plan to Reverse Fatty Liver

I created and followed my new eating plan for 18 months. After 18 months on this plan, I asked my GP for an ultrasound of my liver to check my progress. The tests came back negative; my liver was totally clean without any signs of fat accumulation. Wow, what a relief, and an amazement to my doctor and me! Commitment and determination paid off again. I reversed the non-alcoholic fatty liver. Now I knew that I needed to continue with my eating plan.

I am a living testimonial that when you give your body what it needs, the body has the ability to heal and re-balance itself. When you set your mind to do something, you stay focused and never give up regardless of any obstacles. Once you reverse the fatty liver, it is a commitment for life to continue to follow that eating plan.

Before you start to follow my plan, please consult your doctor because you may have a different medical history and conditions. Your doctor needs to know this to avoid any complications. If you have a Thyroid problem, definitely work with your doctor. I have an underactive Thyroid so it very easy to put on weight.

Again, I made a plan and purchased all the ingredients that I needed on a weekly basis. I placed this list with the plan on my fridge so it was in my vision each time I passed by; a constant reminder to follow it before preparing my meals. Below is the plan I used to reverse non-alcoholic fatty liver. Once the liver is healthy again and to maintain liver health, I reduced the supplements below to only morning and dinner.

First thing in the morning, I:

- Drank a big glass of warm alkaline water with juice of ½ a fresh lemon

- On an empty stomach before breakfast I took 2 tablets of Liver support (Milk Thistle 3500mg, 500mg Globe Artichoke, 500mg Schizandra, 500mg Dandelion, 500mg Taurine). This is an excellent combination to support the liver, and it comes all in one capsule so it is easy to take before a meal.

- Walked 30 to 40 minutes

- On return, I made a fresh vegetable juice (for this you need a juicer that can make juice out of whole vegetables including the skin, because the skin holds a lot of vital nutrients and fiber). Avoid using fruit in juices. Use berries only for antioxidant benefits. Combine and juice:
  - Half cup of fresh or frozen berries or pomegranate
  - 2 tablespoons of fresh oregano leaves or ginger
  - 4 leaves of kale or ½ cup broccoli or ½ cup of rocket greens
  - 1 very small carrot
  - 4 leaves of fresh beetroot or small piece of peeled beetroot
  - 1 cup (or more as needed) of alkaline water

My Breakfast Choices

30 minutes after the juice

- 2 slices of whole meal bread, spread with fresh avocado
  OR
- 1 poached egg on whole meal toast
  OR
- Fresh ricotta cheese drizzled with manuka honey on whole meal toast
  OR
- Whole meal oat organic porridge with water
  OR
- Goat yoghurt with LSA (linseed and almonds) and berries
- Cup of herbal tea (lemongrass & ginger or dandelion & peppermint)

Supplements I choose:

- Omega 3 fatty acids 500mg (good quality), total of 3 per day
- Vitamin D 3, 4000 IU per day (check with your doctor)
- Super anti-oxidant one capsule
- One capsule Super Vitamin C
- One capsule B complex
- 1 good quality of probiotic and prebiotic, taken 30 minutes before meal.

My Morning Tea

- One serve of fresh fruit in season

My Lunch Choices

Supplements - as for breakfast

- Mixed salad with tomatoes, red & yellow capsicum, fresh asparagus, rocket leaves, dandelion leaves or whole artichokes, 100 grams of grilled or boiled chicken or fresh steamed or grilled fish
             OR
- Homemade chicken and vegetable soup
             OR
- Steamed mixed coloured vegetables with a sprinkle of herbs and protein 100 grams (chicken, fish or lamb)

My Afternoon Tea

- Seasonal fresh fruit & ½ cup walnuts (soaked in alkaline water overnight, rinse under alkaline water before you consume them to avoid bloating)

My Dinner Choices

Very small dinner, and before 6pm
Supplements - as for lunch

- Small plate of steamed mixed vegetables
    OR
- Goat yogurt and berries
    OR
- Protein powder mix (pea, brown rice, amaranth) blended with alkaline water
- Peppermint, dandelion or chamomile tea

You can be creative and mix anything healthy, fresh and organic to have more variety. Make your plate look like a rainbow of colour.

Stay away from fatty food, fried food, any pre-packaged food, salt, alcohol, and sugars. Always consult your GP or health professional before you start taking any over the counter medication or natural supplements.

I went to bed between 9 pm and 10 pm, and woke up for my walk between 6 am and 7 am. It is very important to have 8 to 9 hours of good sleep to give your body a chance to rejuvenate and heal itself. If you have anger problems you need to address this because it is directly associated with liver health. If you have sleeping problems, Dr. Vesna can help you with this too as she helped me.

Every day I drank 2 to 3 liters of alkaline water at room temperature to help the body flush out toxins. Meditation or relaxing with music every day for 30 minutes will help your body to heal and rejuvenate itself. This plan worked for me. You may want to ask for help from a professional practitioner to help you.

If you are a healthy person and have a healthy liver, it is important to have an eating plan that supports prevention of ill health and maintains long-term health. If you would like to check the health of your liver, these tests can identify any liver problems:

- blood test to identify elevated liver enzymes
- an ultrasound examination will show any fat accumulation inside and around the liver
- a liver biopsy is the last option.

Your GP can arrange these tests for you.

Chapter 10
How To Achieve Optimal Health Again

Now I would like to share with you, step-by-step, how I recovered from cancer (emotionally, mentally and physically).

My reason for sharing my personal experience with you is to help you. If I can help one person to learn how to stay positive and healthy, and learn how to prevent cancer or how to overcome cancer as I did, it would be a great achievement for me.

What to Avoid to Achieve Optimal Health

Food

- Sugar: avoid sugar as it feeds cancer.
- Processed foods, refined sugars, simple carbohydrate foods, anything made from white flour, artificial flavours and colours, MSG, Aspartame, and trans-fat. Avoid any processed deli meat and hard cheeses, they may contain nitrogen as a preservative, and a lot of salt/sodium.
- Avoid food sprayed with pesticides, and grown with chemical fertilizers. Buy or grow organic food instead.
- Microwave oven: avoid reheating food in plastic containers. If you must use a microwave oven, always use glass or ceramic dishes for reheating food.

Products

- House cleaning chemicals and aero-sprays: avoid pesticides and chemical fertilizers for plants, both in the garden and inside the house. Instead, use organic or eco-friendly products.

- Detergent: avoid ones that contain bleaches, acids, caustic soda and chlorine. Instead, use organic or eco-friendly products.
- Plastic containers and bottles. Only use BPA free ones.
- Hair colours: avoid ones with ammonia, parabens, and other carcinogens.
- Personal care products, including: make-up, skin care, body washes, lotions, shampoo, conditioner, toothpaste, mouthwash, etc. Avoid ones that contain any mineral oils and potentially harmful chemicals (e.g. Propylene glycol - PG, Sodium Laureth Sulfate - SLS, etc.). Always go for more natural options.
- Sun protection. Use organic sun lotion 50+ that is water resistant, and wear protective clothing.
- Avoid Multi-Level Marketing or Direct Selling health/personal care products because their members are trained how to sell their products, and their products only. Unless they are a naturopath, nutritionist or doctor and have training in health and how the body works, their lack of this knowledge can potentially do harm. Trust me because I am talking from personal experience. Always go to a medical doctor or Naturopath/Nutritionist who puts your health first.

Medical

- I decided to avoid too many unnecessary X-Rays, CT scans and mammograms as they contain high radiation levels.
- I also avoided unnecessary medication, alternative medicine/supplements, self-prescribed over the counter medication. Always seek a medical/health professional's advice, and sometimes a second opining is valuable.

Habits

- Avoid smoking, use of alcohol, soft drinks, packaged juices, and pre-packaged canned food.
- Avoid mental and emotional stress, over exercising or over eating, and emotional eating.
- Avoid sitting in front of the TV for too long. Too much exposure to blue light on all digital technology: mobile phone, tablet, TV, computers, etc. I use a blue light protective screen on these.
- Too much sitting or lack of activity can lead to weight or other health challenges. Move regularly, take short breaks, stretch.

How To Clean Your Body

The plan below is beneficial to overcome illness and to support your body to heal, and to become healthy again.

All illness is created by the body's internal system/s being out of balance. Once you bring these systems back into balance, your body starts to heal. Rather than being a one-off task, this it is an ongoing plan to keep your body in healthy balance. You can also implement this plan if you are overweight, underweight or simply for prevention.

1. Brush your body once per week with a dry natural bristle brush before you step into the shower. Always work from your toes up to your heart. This will remove dry skin on a deeper level, and improve your circulation.

2. Every second day in the shower under warm water, exfoliate your body with exfoliating gloves. Always work from your

toes up to your heart to stimulate the lymphatic system and blood flow. Finish your shower with cool water to stimulate circulation. Exfoliation will give your skin a glow, by removing old dead skin cells. It will boost the flow of lymphatic fluids, will help the removal of toxins, and will boost the production of healthy new skin cells.

3. When drying yourself after a shower or bath, always pat your skin with a soft cotton towel, and apply natural lotion to feed your skin. Look for natural botanical oils such as: ivy, birch, coconut oils, almond, rosehip, argon oil or any combination of these. Avoid petrochemicals or any mineral oils as they are potentially carcinogenic and harmful to your health. Anything that you put on your skin is absorbed into your body. Our skin is the largest organ that protects our body, and helps the body to release toxins on a daily basis.

4. Your liver, kidneys, and small and large intestines need to be looked after every day to be able to achieve good health. Focus on organic nutritious food, free from chemicals and pesticides. Eat more cool food to cool your body to avoid internal inflammation e.g. celery, cucumbers, lemons and herbs. Before each meal, eat some fermented food such as: Kimchi, sauerkraut or Kieffer to maintain inner balance of healthy micro-flora and good bacteria. Take milk thistle to help your liver. Eat lots of fresh green vegetables and salads, and healthy proteins such as eggs, turkey, fish, chicken (with skin off), and a variety of beans.

5. Limit red meat to once per week. Avoid processed food such as cakes, soft drinks, simple carbohydrates, trance-fat. Eat more complex carbohydrate food such as: brown rice, brown pasta, quinoa, legumes.

6. Take time out to relax your body and mind.

7. Drink alkaline water and eat a rainbow of colours of fresh fruit and vegetables on a daily basis. Chew slowly, and avoid eating in front of the TV or while reading or using digital devices. Focus and be mindful on your eating.

8. Be active, and go out into nature.

Maintaining Optimal Health

Emotional/Mental Health

- Let go of past emotions, limiting beliefs, physical/emotional/mental stress, emotional traumas. See a professional practitioner to help you address your emotional issues. I can personally recommend Dr. Vesna from Qt.
- Create a healthy environment at home and at work. Create family support that is healthy for all members regardless of age.
- Spend time with family: go for walks or picnics in nature, openly communicate with each other, share how you are feeling, ask for help to support each other.
- Take time out to relax and to rejuvenate your body, mentally, physically and nutritionally.

Nutrition

- Eat healthy organic food, always fresh and free from any additives. Drink water at room temperature. Drink clean alkaline water with a pH level between 7.5 and 8.5.

- Eat food rich in natural minerals, vitamins and antioxidants: dark green leafed organic vegetables, fresh fruit in season, different berries.
- Educate yourself as to how to look after your health. If you need help, ask as it can save your life. Never delay.
- Nourish your body with healthy fresh food. Eat 70% to 80% alkaline food, and 20% to 30% acidic food to keep your body pH in balance. Test your body pH regularly. Your body pH must stay at 7.365 to stay healthy.
- Take natural food-based supplements to support your body. Always seek a medical/health professional's advice, never self-medicate with over-the-counter medicine or natural supplements.
- The nutritional supplements that you may need can be different depending on your health situation and where the cancer is in the body, so avoid going to supermarkets or health food stores and buying anything. Often the sales people are not professional practitioners or cancer experts. You need to see a professional who is trained in integrative medicine and healthy eating. Even better, find a medical doctor that is open minded and practices both conventional and complimentary medicine. Taking supplements is important to support the immune system.
- Always inform your GP what you are taking to ensure it is right for your health.

Daily Habits

- First thing in the morning, start with 200 ml of warm alkaline water. In it, squeeze juice of ½ fresh lemon and drink it slowly.

- Go for a 30-minute walk if you can, increase the time as you feel comfortable.
- Follow with fresh vegetable juice. (You will need a good quality juicer to do nutritional juices that keep nutrients and enzymes alive, including the skin for fiber. Add some alkaline water before blending.) Drink the juice in the first 15 minutes of blending it to preserve the nutritional benefits.

It is very important that you ask for professional advice so you can have the best plan in place: mentally, emotionally, physically and nutritionally.

I was always very concerned about my lifestyle and food choices, especially since I completed my Diplomas in Clinical Nutrition, and Food and Environmental Allergies. After the life-threatening experience, I completely changed my eating plan and my lifestyle. It took a lot of time to do research, and to find what works and what doesn't work. In the end, it was worth it because it helped me to recharge my immune system, and bring my body pH back in balance.

During 2008/9 prior to being diagnosed with cancer, my body was out of balance. My body pH dropped suddenly under 5.0 as I mentioned before. Our body pH needs to be at 7.365 to stay healthy. Regardless how hard I was working to bring my body back in balance and to correct my body pH and level of Vitamin D, it was constantly dropping. At the time of the diagnosis, my Vitamin D blood test showed a low 20, regardless of me taking 2000 IU Vitamin D3 per day. I was very concerned because I know that Vitamin D can protect us against many different cancers. A healthy level of Vitamin D is between 70 and 100.

Vitamin D is fat-soluble and if people take too much, it can be stored in the liver and can create toxicity.

Also, my blood test for ESR showed that inflammation in my body was rising. Anything above 20 is a call for concern. It is necessary to monitor this every 4 to 6 months (as for Vitamin D).

I found that listening to my body and paying attention to changes that occurred over a number of months, and asking my GP questions, definitely saved my life. Because the warning signs were picked up early, this also avoided chemo and radio therapy, painful treatments. No one knows your body as well as you do. This is why it is so important to stay in touch and connected with your body. As we get busier in life we can neglect and ignore that vital connection between body and mind (as Dr Vesna explains in chapter 1 of this book). As soon as you notice changes happening in your body, even if it is a false alarm, go to your GP and check it out.

Make a commitment to yourself. I need to mention that I was prepared to do whatever was necessary to get well again. Now this is very important; you need to be committed to make the necessary changes, and to follow the plan for the rest of your life. You may need professional help to make changes, and to continue with the plan. It is worthless to start making changes and then when you have a challenge, to give up. You are giving yourself permission to fail, and you are playing yoyo with your health.

Avoid getting discouraged if you find that changes are happening slowly. Remember, that your body needs to rebuild itself in order to heal, and to conquer daily challenges. As you may know our body has over 70 trillion cells. All of them need to receive nutrients every day to support our body to stay healthy, and to work in harmony with each other to rejuvenate our body for optimal health. Start with small changes, then each week add one or two things until you have a complete plan in place.

ASK FOR HELP!

I asked for help from a well experienced Clinical Hypnotherapist who holds a PhD qualification in the field. Dr Vesna from Qt helped me to address the emotional issues and trauma that I was holding onto from childhood, and bullying during my life. That alone has made a big difference in how I dealt with the healing process. It was challenging to work on emotions because I had suppressed them unconsciously for so long. It was so important for me to address these emotions as suppressed emotions were detrimental to my health.

My GP was excellent; she was supportive, educational and kept me on track with all the tests that were necessary to monitor my progress for recovery. I also asked for help from a Naturopath that practiced Chinese Medicine as a back up to see how my body is healing and repairing at a cellular level. Illness can leave behind cellular memory, and cellular memory can trigger the illness to return. For that reason, I worked with Dr Vesna on the emotional issues to eliminate those cellular memories. She is well educated and very passionate in helping people to address these issues.

Ask for help and support from your family and friends, and create a stress-free environment at home and at work. If you are not ready for heavy work, ask your employer for lighter duties until you fully recover.

How I made positive lifestyle changes: mental, emotional, physical and nutritional.

1.   I already had a water purifier in the house. When I tested it, it was producing acidic water. I did a bit of research for different filters to give me more alkaline water. Now my whole family is drinking healthy water. Water is the most important nutrient that the body needs to start to heal, and to stay healty. Alkaline water flushes out acid and waste from our body, and helps to keep our body hydrated at a cellular level. If the water is too acidic, it is unable to go into our organs and cells. This leaves our body dehydrated and acidic. Water needs to be structured in very small clusters to be able to enter the cells.

2.   I started to do exercise that I enjoy doing, and that was beneficial for me. Soon after I woke up, I put on my walking shoes. I was walking every day for 30 to 40 minutes, regardless of the weather. Every second day, I used an Infra bed and bio blanket for 1 hour to help my body improve circulation, and help the lymphatic system to flow more effectively.

3.   Relax. Take time out to relax. I relax after lunch, either meditation or just simply listening to relaxing music.

4.   Support. Have supportive people around you, open up to them. Avoid bottling up your emotions, as this can create another health issue. Be there for each other, express your thoughts, share your life experiences with each other. Have conversations over a cup of tea or simply a glass of water.

5.   The nutrition plan took a bit longer to go through because what consciously sounds right may need a bit of testing

and experimenting. Your body will let you know what is right for you, and what you need to avoid. There are some books that suggest that one plan fits all. We are all individuals, and unique and each person responds differently to the same foods and nutritional supplements.

I was very vigilant about what I chose, what gave me benefits, and what was not agreeing with me. I had a notebook, and each day I wrote down what was good for me and what was disagreeing with me. What was disagreeing with me I stopped consuming for four months, and then I started to introduce these back into my eating plan one by one. I was very passionately observing what was happening. That is how to eliminate any food allergies.

The nutrition plan needed to include a variety of healthy organic foods to help the body to repair and heal itself. I started with what I call the "Rainbow of Colours" healthy eating plan.

Rainbow of Colours Healthy Eating Plan

- A variety of 2-3 fresh fruits per day, fruit that is rich in antioxidants and phytonutrients (also known as "Super Nutrients"). All berries are good, red grapes with skin and seeds, goji, acacia, pomegranate, apples and pears, stone fruit when in season.
- Fresh vegetables: approximately 7 to 9 serves per day (one serve is equal to a ½ cup). More green leafed vegetables, and less root vegetables.
- Good complex carbohydrates (2 serves per day). For example: 2 slices of whole meal bread or pita/flat bread or whole meal pasta or brown rice or quinoa.

- Good organic, free range protein: 10 grams per 1 kilogram of body weight per day. This means if you weigh 60 kilos, you need to have 60 grams of protein per day. For example: fish, turkey, chicken, lamb, beef. Limit beef and lamb to only once per week.
- Use goat cheese, yoghourt and milk instead of cow products, particularly if you are dairy intolerant. Many dairy intolerant people can tolerate goat products.
- Avoid powder protein as it may contain hidden preservatives, chemicals, synthetic hormones and steroids.
- Brown and red lentils, beans and split pea.
- Red and green salads. Bitter leaves such as dandelion and rocket are good to clean toxins out of the liver.
- In the first two years after surgery, I avoided all sugary foods. Now for special occasions, I have a very small piece of cake so that I can control how much fat and sugar I consume. I made these myself – you will find some of my favourite recipes in Chapter 14 of this book.
- Avoid take away food, frozen prepared foods and tinned foods.

Plenty of Healthy Fluids

- Start the day with ½ lemon squeezed in warm water to give your digestive system a boost, and to help the liver to break down fat.
- Follow with fresh vegetable juice. This is a big help to get more nutrients to your system, and it is very beneficial to add green powder, fibre and digestive enzymes to the juice. Sip the juice slowly to mix the enzymes with your saliva.

- Drink 2-3-litres of alkaline water at room temperature per day to flush out acid and toxins out of the system. Peppermint or ginger tea aids digestion. Chamomile tea before bedtime helps you to relax, and to have a good night sleep of 8 to 9 hours. Green tea has valuable antioxidants. During wintertime, drink Echinacea tea to boost the immune system.
- Avoid any alcohol and soft drinks. Have one cup of good quality expresso coffee before lunch if you desire. Avoid drinking coffee after 3pm as it can interfere with your sleep.

Planning and Support

- Like I said earlier, this is very important and needs time to plan. Take each day slowly, avoid stress. If you need help, find a practitioner that is interested in helping you to reach your health goal. The practitioner needs to put your needs first, to listen to you and understand you because we are all unique and need specific attention; <u>one size does not fit all</u>.
- If you are taking supplements or medication avoid taking these with tea or coffee because it could interfere with their absorption. With prescription medication, always follow your doctor's or pharmacist's advice. Never use alcohol with medication.

Cut Down Processed Sugar - Understanding GI and GL Glycemic Index (GI) and Glycemic Load (GL)

What is the GI?

The GI is one the best tools for fat loss. It measures how quickly foods break down into sugars in your bloodstream. High glycemic foods turn into blood sugar very quickly. Starchy foods like potatoes are a good example. Potatoes have such a high GI rating, it's almost the same as eating raw sugar. Other high GI foods include: all highly processed foods, simple carbohydrates (e.g. white bread, pasta, rice, cakes, biscuits, pastries, etc.).

What is the difference between the Glycemic Index (GI) and Glycemic Load (GL)?

- The GI tells you how quickly foods spike your blood sugar; it won't tell you how much carbohydrates you are getting per serve.
- Glycemic Load (GL) is a great help especially for people who have a weight problem or are diabetics. It measures the amounts of carbohydrates in each serve of food.

Food with a GL under 10 is a good choice for carbohydrates. Food that falls between 10 and 20 on the GL scale has a moderate effect on your blood sugar. Food with a GL above 20 will cause blood sugar and insulin spikes. If you do choose foods above 20 GL, it is best to eat them in very small portions, and only occasionally.

Foods that have a GL 0 to 10 are:

- Broccoli, Cabbage, Celery, Cauliflower, Green beans, Spinach and all vegetables that grow green leaves above ground.

- Mushrooms, Almonds, Hazelnuts, Macadamia nuts, Pecan nuts, Walnuts

- Lean organic grass-fed Beef, Chicken, Eggs, Fish, Lamb, Pork, Veal, Deer/Venison, Buffalo, Rabbit, Duck, Ostrich, Shellfish, Lobster, and Turkey

Avoid any bought juices as they are high in artificial sugars and preservatives.

By following the GI & GL it will help you to cut down processed sugar. Good books to assist you are "The New Glucose Revolution", and "Complete Guide to GI Values A to Z Food Categories for Optimal Health." The second book is for people with diabetes. Any good book store will have these books.

Chapter 11
Water and Your Health

Water is not just another substance - it is the life force of nature. Therefore, we cannot live without water. If our body is deprived of water for a long period of time, the body becomes toxic and our life can come to an end.

Good quality, clean alkaline water is the most important nutrient that our body needs for good health in the long term. Water is needed to cleanse our body (both outside and inside) of toxins and waste every day. It nourishes our cells and keeps our skin nice and plump, and moist. Water also replenishes our body from the loss of fluids during illness, perspiration, heat in summer, dry winds and cold weather during winter.

We need quality water to maintain our personal hygiene, and for cooking our meals. Water needs to be free from chemicals and pesticides; elements that are damaging to our health. Water needs to be between 7.5 pH and 8 pH. Anything under 7.5 pH is too acidic. Over acidic water can bring imbalance to our body, can cause inflammation and arthritis, and can weaken our bones. Water with a pH of 8 to 9 is best used for short periods of time by people with severe illnesses, until the body is brought back into balance. Otherwise, over alkaline water can be as damaging to our body as over acidic water.

Water needs to be clean and free from any contamination. For example, rain water is no longer as clean as it was many decades ago. As rain falls it passes through layers and layers of industrial pollution: through the pollution in the clouds, in the air, on our roof, and into water tanks. Therefore, it is important that you use appropriate filters to eliminate toxins and algae that may accumulate in stored water.

A large number of people are under the wrong impression that bottled water is healthy. It could be treated with chemicals that are harmful for humans. It gets more confusing with so many water purifier machines and different units, and sales people pushing to sell and some giving false information.

When I started to look for water units, I admit that I too was fooled with pushy sales people more than once. Once I educated myself through research about good water purifier units, I started to ask questions that most sales people could not answer. Some even rudely brushed me off as if I did not know what I was talking about. It is that attitude that gave me more power to do even further research about pH levels, and the effect unhealthy water has on our body.

Tap water is unhealthy because it is treated with many different additives. Many individuals are possibly allergic to these which can create more health problems. Just look at fluoride. There are topical and systemic made fluorides. Topical fluorides are used by dentists as a gel, applied to our teeth to prevent tooth decay. The fluoride added to toothpaste is purified Sodium Fluoride, systemic fluoride. There is even a warning on the packaging that it should not be swallowed.

Systemic fluoride is Hydrofluorosilic Acid (S 7 class 8 corrosive). This form of fluoride when added to water as a water treatment ends up in our food, juices, bread, baby formulas and practically in every food item that we consume. It is a corrosive chemical that is ingested systemically that can damage fertility, bones (e.g. Arthritis and hip fractures in elderly), brain, lower the IQ, affect the Pineal gland and Thyroid function. When water treated with fluoride is boiled, it further increases the fluoride levels.

Many independent scientists, doctors, dentists and other health professionals oppose fluoridation. As at November 2018, over 4,000 professionals have supported and signed a statement to end water fluoridation worldwide. Also, as at May 2019, 98% of western European countries' population drank non fluoridated water. Despite this, tooth decay rates have declined in Europe to the same extent as those in fluoridated countries.

Chlorine added to water is another chemical that has potential health concerns. Many people are allergic to it. If after a shower you experience itching skin, and your skin starts to flake that is the effect of chlorine. Water filters need to be able to filter out chlorine, and all harmful substances in the water. Please do your own research to check your water quality.

Understanding your body chemical balance acidity and alkalinity

When we are born, we are full of alkaline reserves and our metabolism moves smoothly leaving our body balanced. When it comes to health, balance is everything. The balance of acids and alkalis is essential for good health and survival - it creates the body pH. What is pH? It stands for potential hydrogens, and it measures how acidic or alkaline our internal body fluids are. These include: our blood, saliva, urine, our gastrointestinal tract and fluids.

Albert Szent-Gyorgyi (a Hungarian biochemist, Nobel Laureate in Physiology and Medicine in 1937, and discoverer of vitamin C) once noted "The body is alkaline by design, but acidic by function."

Here is your guideline for a healthy body pH.

- From 0 to 6.5 is acidic
- From 6.75 to 7.365 is normal
- From 7.37 to 14 is over alkaline

An over alkaline and an over acidic body are both equally a health concern.

The pH of Selected Body Tissue:

- 7.8 - 8.0 = Pancreatic juices (upper small intestine)
- 7.35 - 7.45 = Blood
- 6.9 = Liver
- 6.8 - 7.4 = Saliva (mouth)
- 5.6 - 8.0 = Duodenum
- 6.0 - 7.5 = Small intestine
- 5.5 - 7.0 = Colon
- 6.1 = Muscle
- 4.5 - 8.0 = Urine
- 1.5 - 2.0 = Stomach Acid

As you can see, different organs function at different optimal pH levels. The body maintains pH levels using the body's primary systems:
- buffer system using digestive and systematic enzymes
- respiratory control using breathing and lungs to maintain optimal levels of oxygen
- renal using kidneys to eliminate acid and toxins with urine and faeces,

- lymphatic system to bring nutrients to the body, and eliminate toxins and waste out of the body tissue and blood.

Alkalinity depends on health, longevity and quality of life. People with illnesses such as: arthritis, diabetes, pain, cancer, inflammation, etc. are acidic. Unless they make changes to correct the body's pH levels, illnesses will turn chronic. Body tissue when too acidic, and if not neutralized or eliminated, has a long list of harmful effects upon the body.

It is important that you understand that you need to monitor your acid/alkaline levels. When these are out of balance in small proportion, it is easier to correct than when the gaps are big.

In addition to people with illness, people who also have higher acidity in their bodies are those who consume junk food, smoke, drink alcohol, have a diet high in animal protein, eat fatty foods and poor selection of vegetables. People with unresolved emotional issues, with very high stress level, or who work in polluted environments are more acidic. If you are concerned about your pH level and your health, find a practitioner who specializes in balancing and testing body pH levels.

If you wish to educate yourself on pH levels, there are books written by doctors listed in the appendix at the back of this book.

How to balance your body pH

What do you need to do to balance your pH levels? First, test your pH levels to determine their current levels. Then this is what I recommend to adjust the pH level:

1. A water unit to produce alkaline water pH of 8 to 9 to rebalance body pH, then water pH of 7.5 to 8 to maintain optimal health. Avoid falling into the trap of sales people pushing expensive units. You can purchase an alkaline water unit starting from as little as $220 to $800 depending on the size of the unit. Consider whether you need a portable or a fixed under kitchen bench unit. Before you buy a unit, ask them to test the water pH level.

2. Instead of the above water units, you can have a whole house water treatment. This will give you clean water at every tap in the house. It could cost you from $2,600 including installation of the unit.

3. To keep the water unit producing alkaline water, you need to change the filters regularly. The frequency depends on the unit and the manufacturer's recommendations.

4. Plan your eating with 80% alkaline, and 20% acidic foods. Please refer below for a guide.

5. Change your daily eating plan to 5 smaller meals per day. Make breakfast and lunch bigger portions, with dinner and snacks being smaller.

6. Eliminate all soft drinks and, if possible, alcohol from your lifestyle. Drink alkaline water only.

7. If you are a smoker, stop smoking.

8. Manage your stress and emotions.

9. Manage your weight and emotional eating.

10. If you are buying takeaway food, always choose from healthier food outlets.

11. Plan exercise that you enjoy every day. Avoid over doing it.

How to balance your body alkalinity with food
List of Alkaline foods - consume these 80% of your daily food intake

Vegetables:
Artichokes, Asparagus, Beets, Peppers yellow/red, Bok Choy, Broccoli, Brussel Sprouts, Cabbage, Carrots, Cauliflower, Celery, Chard, Chicory, Collards, Cucumbers, Eggplant, Endives, Garlic, Greens, Jerusalem Artichokes, Kale, Kelp, Kohlrabi, Leek, Lettuce, Mushrooms (all), Mustard Greens, Okra, Olives ripe, Onion (all), Parsley, Parsnips, Peas (fresh), Pumpkin, Radish, Seaweed, Spinach, Spirulina, Sprouts (all), Squash (all), Tomatoes, Turnips, Watercress, Wheat Grass, Zucchini

Cereals and Grains:
Amaranth, Barley Grass, Millet, Spelt

Fresh Fruit:
Apple, Apricot, Avocado, Banana, Berries, Cantaloupe, Cherries, Coconut, Currants, Dates, Figs, Grapefruit, Grapes, Lemon, Lime, Melons, Nectarine, Orange, Peach, Pear, Pineapple, Plums, Tangerine, Tropical Fruits, Watermelon

Beverages:
Alkaline Water, Apple Cider Vinegar, Dandelion Tea, Fresh Vegetable Juices, Green Tea, Ginseng Tea, Green Juices, Herbal Tea

Nuts and seeds (natural):
Almonds, Chestnuts, Flax Seeds (ground), Pumpkin Seeds, Sesame Seeds, Sprouted Seeds, Sunflower Seeds, Walnuts

Protein:
Beans, Tempeh, Tofu

Sweeteners:
Stevia or Monk Fruit

Spices and Seasonings:
All herbs (fresh and dry), Chili Peppers, Cinnamon, Cumin, Curry, Dill, Fennel, Ginger, Horseradish, Mustard, Olive Oil, Sea Salt (unprocessed).

List of Acidic foods: consume these 20% of your daily food intake

Meat, poultry and seafood:
Beef, Buffalo, Chicken, Clams, Crab, Duck, Geese, Lamb, Lobster, Mussels, Mutton, Pork, Quail, Rabbit, Red Snapper, Salmon, Sardines, Scallops, Tuna, Turkey, Veal, Venison

Condiments:
Dressings (packaged), Jams, Jellies, Ketchup/Tomato Sauce, Mayonnaise, Mustard, Olives, Peanut Butter, Soy Sauce, Tahini, Vinegar

Breads and Flours:
Cereals in general, Processed Corn, Cornmeal, Cornstarch, Wheat and Rye products, All processed white products (cakes, pasta, bread, etc.)

Fats and Oils:
Avocado oil, Canola oil, Corn oil, Flax oil, Lard, Margarine, Safflower oil, Sesame oil, Sunflower oil, Vegetable oil

Beverages:
Beer, Black Tea, Coffee, Hard Liquor, Processed Juices, Soft Drinks, Sport Drinks, Wine

Fruit and Vegetables:
Artificially dried, roasted, sweetened - all fruit and vegetables, Canned Fruit, Canned Olives, Canned Vegetables, Cranberries, Glazed Fruit, Pickled Fruit, Preserved Fruit and Vegetables, Processed Vegetables

Nuts and Seeds:
Brazil nuts, Cashew nuts, Peanuts, Pecans, Roasted nuts, Salted nuts

Grains and Legumes:
Barley, All Dry Beans, Cumquat, Lentils, All Processed Rice, Rice Cakes and Rice Milk, Rolled Oats, Soybeans, Soymilk, Wheat

Dairy Products:
All processed cheeses and dairy processed products, Eggs and Egg processed products

Sweets:
Artificial sweeteners, Cakes, Chocolates, All biscuits, Doughnuts, Pies, Corn Syrup, Sugar

OTHER:
Distilled Vinegar, Potatoes, Wheat Germ.

Chapter 12
Your Digestive System

How well your digestive system works is a reflection of how you feel and how healthy you are, because good health starts in the digestive system. It is important to be aware that our digestive system starts in our mouth and ends at the anus. Depending on what we are eating, it takes approximately 4 to 8 hours for food to be digested and eliminated. As soon as we start to think about food, saliva starts to release digestive enzymes in our mouth. How well we chew our food also affects our digestive health. Here are some steps to follow to avoid digestive problems.

1. Eat slowly and in a relaxing environment. Avoid watching TV or reading while you are eating.

2. Avoid eating when you are angry, frustrated or afraid as it affects acidity in the stomach, and your liver becomes affected.

3. Eliminate from your eating plan: fried foods, refined sugars, simple carbohydrates (white bread, white pasta, white rice, white potatoes, etc.)

4. Cut down dairy products because they produce mucus build up and block respiratory passages. Goat products and products made from rice milk are fine.

5. Limit coffee to one per day, and instead drink good quality water, black tea, green tea or herbal tea.

6. Limit alcohol and bought juices that contain artificial sugars and possible preservatives because they block the absorption of iron, minerals and vitamins from food.

7. Chew every bite until you feel liquid in your mouth. Allow your saliva to do its job to avoid unpleasant indigestion, gas and bloating.

8. Avoid drinking any liquid with food. If you need to take medication with food, only sip a small amount of room temperature water. If you drink while eating or drink very hot fluids while eating, this can interrupt the intestine flora and digestive enzymes.

9. Eat fruit as a snack away from the meal. It is best to have snacks for morning tea or afternoon tea.

10. Stop smoking and consuming alcohol.

11. Have your dinner meal 3 hours before bedtime to have an uninterrupted good night's sleep. Plan your dinner meal to be light and smaller portions for easier digestion.

12. When possible, go to bed no later than 9.30pm because our body rejuvenates itself before midnight.

13. At any time you start to feel indigestion/acid reflux/gas/bloating, before you reach for antacid tablets, STOP and find out what is the cause of the problem. Address the problem with natural remedies such as peppermint or fennel tea. You can obtain peppermint essence at the chemist. Take 50 mils of hot water, add 5 drops of essence and drink it. Sit down in a reclined position and massage

your stomach in clockwise movements. To avoid these problems in the future, increase enzyme foods in you eating plan, including:

- Pineapple for bromalin enzyme
- Papaya for papine enzyme
- Raw fruit for Betaine Hydrochloride or take digestive enzymes in powder form made from fruit and vegetables
- Avoid over cooked vegetables as this can destroy enzymes. To keep natural enzymes at their best, steam or stir-fry vegetables so they are less than half way cooked. Eat a variety of colours of vegetables in a raw unprocessed state.

If you have a digestive problem, even if you are eating healthy, it would be wise to check yourself for food allergies or sensitivities, irritable bowel syndrome (IBS), Celiac or Candida Albicans (known as a yeast overgrowth or yeast infection). If you are experiencing any of the above, you need to work with a professional health practitioner and/or medical practitioner to bring it under control, follow a specific eating plan, and take appropriate medication/supplements to rebuild your digestive system.

You need to have regular bowel movement, at least once per day. If you are having problems with constipation, re-evaluate your eating plan and make adjustments without laxatives. Have more soluble and insoluble fiber in your eating plan. Organic Aloe Vera, prunes, natural fiber with lots of alkaline water can help to keep you regular. It may help to place 3 dry figs in a glass, top them with alkaline water, leave overnight to soak. The next morning, eat the soaked figs and drink the water they were soaked in too. If that does not help, seek professional advice. Avoid laxatives because your body can become dependent on these, and they can damage the gut flora.

Where to find soluble fiber?

Soluble fiber is found in foods such as: oat bran, barley, nuts, seeds, beans, lentils, fruit (citrus, apples, strawberries), and many vegetables.

Where to find Insoluble fiber?

Insoluble fiber is found in foods such as: whole wheat, whole grain products, vegetables and wheat bran.

Just to be healthy we need 30 grams of fiber every day. For optimal health and prevention, we need about 75 grams of fiber a day. Fiber needs to be supported with enough fluids. Alkaline water is the best; it will help to flush waste and toxins out of the system so that it is able to work effectively. If you have fiber and not enough water, you may become constipated.

If you are given antibiotics by your doctor, always take these with prebiotics & probiotics to protect your gut flora. Antibiotics disrupt the gut bacteria and impact bone health which can lead to osteoporosis. "The research in the American Journal of Pathology has published that antibiotics could disrupt gut microbiota and causes a Pro-inflammatory response that affects the process of releasing of minerals that are important for bone health".

Because we are exposed to polluted and damaging substances on a daily basis, every day we need to take prebiotics and probiotics to assist our digestive system, and to protect and keep our gut flora healthy. Avoid drinking coffee and tea with food, because it interrupts iron absorption. Educate yourself on gut health. There are a number of books available on gut health, a few are mentioned in the appendix at the back of this book.

The Immune System

The immune system is one of the most remarkable and complex systems within the human body. It has the ability to produce millions of specific antibodies within a minute, and to recognize and disarm billions of different invaders/antigens. It makes sense to keep the immune system strong so we have the optimal ability to protect our health.

The immune system is made of: Lymph nodes, Thymus, Liver, Spleen, Skin, Bone marrow, B cells and antibodies, T cells and Macrophages and Monocytes.

For a healthy immune system, nutritional support is necessary, and it is important to avoid unnecessary stress. Over exercising suppresses the immune system. Diets high in animal protein and saturated fats can clog up the lymphatic vessels.

How to strengthen your immune system?

Your immune strength is totally dependent on: an optimal nutritional healthy eating plan, food-based vitamins and minerals, good mental and emotional health, and a toxic free environment.

1. Well-balanced healthy eating plans comprise of: low-fat, 20% protein, 20% complex carbohydrates, and 60% fresh vegetables, fruit, seeds and nuts. Always buy organic food

or direct from the farmer as you will get better nutritional value than from supermarkets (where fruit and vegetables are stored in cool rooms for long periods of time before they reach the supermarket shelves. By that time most of the vital nutritional value is lost.).

2. Prebiotics and probiotics are necessary to protect gut health, and keep the immune system strong.

3. Antioxidants are needed to fight free radicals. These include: Vitamins E, A, D, Resveratrol, Astaxanthin, Iron, Selenium, Zinc, B1, B2, B6, B12 and Folic Acid. C–Super formula in powder form. Use supplements under professional supervision for best results.

4. Alkaline water to help flush toxins and waste out of the system, and to keep our internal body hydrated.

5. Emotional issues can affect the immune system on so many levels, including suppressing the immune system. It is very important to address all emotional issues, limiting beliefs, etc. to help your immune system protect your body.

Inflammation – The Internal Silent Killer

There are two types of inflammation:

1. Acute: as a result of scratches, cuts, bruises, injuries – the body naturally heals those.

2. Chronic inflammation is referred to as a silent killer because it can be undetected for many years, and in the process cause damage to internal organs and tissue. The biggest factors contributing to chronic inflammation are poor food choices, excess weight, cigarette smoke, UV radiation, stress, emotional issues and toxic environments.

The good news is that we can measure internal inflammation with a simple blood test.

- The CRP count needs to be under 4. If it is above 4 it shows infection in the body.
- The ESR count needs to be under 20. If it is above 20 it shows inflammation in the body.

Chronic inflammation can slowly spread and lead to serious metabolic breakdown, with big effects for your long-term health. This includes health conditions like: rheumatoid arthritis, inflammatory bowel disease, eczema, obesity, diabetes, atherosclerosis, high blood pressure, Alzheimer's, osteoporosis, cancer, depression and many other health issues. Please work with a medical/health professional to address chronic inflammation.

How to prevent or reduce internal chronic inflammation

Preventing chronic inflammation is not an overnight fix; it requires ongoing care of your health. To address chronic inflammation, first you need to find its root cause. Then you need to make lifestyle changes, and adhere to a good healthy eating plan. There are foods that cause inflammation, and foods that soothe inflammation.

Food that causes inflammation includes:
- Processed and sugary foods
- Trans fats and vegetable shortening: which are present in a variety of snack foods, fried foods, baked foods, heated, dried, pasteurized, smoked and charcoal grilled foods.

In addition to diet, certain life choices may contribute to inflammation. Also environmental toxicity from water, air, food pollutants and heavy metals. Avoid alcohol, coffee, cigarettes, stimulants, medication (prescribed and over the counter – always discuss any medication with your doctor before making any changes). Sleep deprivation, being overweight or obese, diabetes, an existing heart condition, and constant psychological, emotional and physical stress can all contribute to chronic inflammation.

Food that helps reduce inflammation includes:
- Citrus fruit, tomatoes, wild salmon, dark leafy greens, broccoli, and cabbage.
- Herbs which also have antioxidant benefits include: ginger, parsley, cardamon, turmeric, rosemary, thyme, oregano and cumin.
- Berries, olive oil, omega-3 oils, seeds, raw cacao, alkaline water, raw activated nuts (soak nuts overnight in alkaline water, drain water in the morning, peel the skin off the nuts before you eat them).

Other lifestyle changes which will help with reducing inflammation include:
- Supplements that help with inflammation are: Folic acid-B complex, Vitamin D, C, A, E, antioxidants, multi vitamins and minerals.
- Detoxify your body regularly and naturally with healthy eating, a lot of green fresh vegetables and fresh vegetable juices in the morning. Add to juices: fresh ginger, mint, coriander, 1/2 whole lemon. Avoid using pre-packaged detox products over the long term as they can potentially cause health problems.

- Reduce stress: work on your emotional issues, reduce toxins in your home and at the work place.
- Have a good night's sleep, 7-8 hours.
- Gentle walking every day in nature.
- Meditation, Yoga and relaxation to music.

Chapter 13
Cancer and Life After Cancer

This is probably the most feared word that we as human dread to hear. For people who are from a family that has a long history of cancer, they hope that it won't affect them. Coming from a family without a history of cancer, and following a healthy lifestyle and healthy eating plan, you definitely believe that you will avoid it.

Living in the 21st century surrounded with much technology, exposed to toxic environments, and the lower quality of food in supermarkets, it is more challenging to estimate what could happen. I believe that emotional issues, an over stressed society, overindulgence in alcohol and recreational substances, environmental toxics, and over processed unhealthy fast food, have a major effect on the body's health. Having said that, I for one come from a family without a cancer history, never smoked, never consumed alcohol or took recreational substances.

However, for a number of years I was under stress, had many emotional issues from the past, and coming from a European ancestry we are known for eating a lot of animal protein and very rich food choices. I was on prescribed HRT for 9 years. By the time I educated myself in healthier options, the above had already started to cause damage on a cellular level.

Looking back on my life before cancer, I was very much focused on achieving a good living for my family and my relatives. I never asked what I wanted for myself. I never had time to relax. I was always on the go, looking after everyone except myself. I had my first holiday ever after working for 30 years. Returning from the holiday, I felt guilty to be away for 3 months on my own.

Being diagnosed with cancer gave me the shock of my life. It gave me a different perspective about what is important in life, and what is unnecessary to worry about. I learned during all this madness that stressing about something that is out of my control is pointless. That was the biggest lesson that helped me to turn my life around. I decided to focus on the future, and on things that I can control. I reminded myself of my mottos that "prevention is better than cure", and that "a healthy person has many wishes, a sick person has only one, to be healthy."

I live my life by my beliefs and values. I appreciate every day that has been given to me, and value everything in my life regardless of how small or big it may be. I value people in my life, and I am grateful for everything that I was given and that I have achieved in my life. I acknowledge the people in my life. I like to be an example to people who may be confused and who may need direction; to help them to look after themself and live a healthier and more fulfilled life.

My personal experience has taught me that to overcome cancer or any other illness it is important to follow these 10 steps:

1. Follow a healthy nutritional eating plan
2. Drink alkaline clean water
3. Detox naturally
4. Maintain a strong immune system (white blood cells & lymphatic system)
5. Have a positive attitude and address your emotions
6. Make lifestyle changes e.g. adequate sleep, sunlight, exercise

7. Ensure oxygen is delivered to your cells via alkaline food

8. Have a toxic free, clean environment

9. Use only 100% organic feminine hygiene pads and organic nappies for babies

10. See your medical/health professional, have tests and a health assessment once per year to have peace of mind, and early detection of any abnormalities. I do the following tests:

- Blood pressure
- Blood sugar for diabetes
- Cholesterol test
- Thyroid test T3, T4, TSH, PTH
- Ovarian cancer CA 125
- CRP for infection and Cancer
- ESR for body inflammation
- Complete hormone tests
- FBT (full blood test with Iron studies B12, Folate, Vitamin D)
- Bowel cancer test
- Breast screening
- Homocystine levels
- Bone screening (DEXA test)
- Any others that your GP may feel is necessary.

My life after cancer

As I am writing these pages, it has been 14 years since I had the surgery. In 2025, I will be celebrating my 80th birthday. I am very happy to share with my readers this good news because it has been a grueling first 5 years. Each time that I needed to go for a check-up, I needed to use all my energy to think positively and avoid stressing. Most difficult was every time I arrived at the hospital waiting room, and seeing all the unfortunate women with fear across their faces as they waited for their examinations or test results not knowing what to expect.

It is a constant reminder that we need to be kind to each other, and to appreciate what we have in life. I believe that we as women have a lot to offer society, and we need to educate each other and share our experiences, both good and not so good. I learned that by being positive it is much easier to go through challenging situations, and to be an example to people who need extra support.

One would think that after 5 years of battling cancer and getting excellent results and winning, that you deserve a rest. Wrong - as I mentioned life is full of surprises. On 16th February 2014 I fell and crushed my left ankle and tibia, simply by slipping on some dry leaves during a walk in nature. The surgeon commented that the break was worse than he had seen in the worst motor bike accident. I ended up in emergency, followed by a double surgery, agonizing pain and struggling for the next six months on crutches. This put my whole body structure out of balance.

After the hysterectomy, the doctor and oncologist left me without an explanation or advice as to how to protect my bones from density loss. As I learned during my research, hormonal imbalance can create enormous health issues, including bone loss. I remember when I was on HRT, doctors were telling women that estrogen will protect us from bone loss.

New research shows that progesterone is more important for protection against bone loss. In their books, Dr. J. Lee, Dr. Jonatan V. Wright, MD and Lane Lenard, PhD, explain in detail the benefits of bio-identical hormone replacement therapy.

These are excellent reading, and are very educational. You will find the details of their books in the appendix at the back of this book.

Here is a very important message to all women that have had their ovaries removed. Ask your doctor for advice as to how to protect yourself from bone loss. Because once you have removed your ovaries, your body does not produce enough of the hormones (estrogen and progesterone) to protect you from developing osteoporosis. With that comes another problem. If you have breast cancer or cancer in any reproductive organ, you may need to stay away from HRT, and any foods that produce estrogen (e.g. soy products). Please speak to your medical/health professional about your specific situation.

For many years, I had a DEXA scan for bone density every 2 years. Prior to 2008, I had a good reading with only a 2% loss of bone density in 2 years. Once I was diagnosed with cancer, I put all my focus on beating cancer, and I totally forgot to do a DEXA scan for a number of years. During my ankle and leg surgery recovery, I did a lot of research about what could cause such a bad bone breakage from a simple slip on flat ground.

As I mentioned before, when women's ovaries are removed the body does not produce enough of the hormones estrogen and progesterone to support bone density.   That can lead to developing osteoporosis. Once I was able to start walking with crutches, I went to do a DEXA scan. I was devastated to learn that I had lost 35% of my bone density over 5 years. Now I understand why I broke my leg so easily, and why my recovery was so slow. To this day, over 10 years later, I still cannot walk and balance my body without the help of a walking stick.

How to keep your bones strong and avoid developing osteoporosis

Your GP may suggest medication to prevent osteoporosis. I chose not to take medication. Instead, I developed a specific program for myself. According to Dr. Rath's Cellular Research Centre, micronutrient vitamins plus amino acids are needed to protect and strengthen bones, combined with a healthy eating plan. It is also important to avoid smoking and alcohol as these deplete the micronutrients in the body. I use the following to strengthen my bones:

- Supplements: Calcium, Vitamin D, Vitamin C, Vitamin E, Vitamin A, Vitamin K2, plus Folic Acid
- Micronutrients: Magnesium, Manganese, Potassium, Zinc, Baron, Iodine, Silica.

Calcium and Vitamin D are very important for bone strength.

How to test Vitamin D levels

Avoid taking Vitamin D supplements before you consult your GP and have a blood test, because Vitamin D is toxic if overdosed. It is fat soluble and is stored in the liver. Make an appointment with your GP and ask for the blood test. Your GP will send you to Pathology for the test. It usually takes 3-4 days for the test results to come to your GP. Your GP will then advise if you need to supplement and how much, and if and when you are required to repeat the blood test. That will give you peace of mind.

Keep in mind that an appropriate level of Vitamin D is vital because it has been scientifically shown that it can prevent a number of different cancers. A healthy level of Vitamin D is 70 to 90, especially if you have a history of cancer. You will need to be monitored by your GP to avoid accumulation of Vitamin D in the liver - that can become toxic, and create health issues. Vitamin D3 is better than D2.

Chapter 14
Recipes for Prevention, Recovery and Rejuvenation of the Body

I created the recipes in this chapter purposefully for my recovery journey. You may choose to use these to help you to: prevent ill health, to heal your body at a cellular level, to strengthen your immune defenses, and to rejuvenate your body to be healthier and stronger in the future.

Herbs and spices in your kitchen

For centuries, herbs and spices have been in use for culinary and medicinal purposes. More and more of the population is now also using herbs and spices for culinary, medicinal and therapeutic purposes. They are especially used for various chronic conditions. There is now ample evidence that spices and herbs possess antioxidants, anti-inflammatory, anticarcinogenic, and glucose and cholesterol-lowering benefits. They also enhance cognition and moods. You will find more information on the health benefits of herbs and spices at the National Library of Medicine.

As a child, I grew up learning about herbs from my grandmother. When I was in primary school, we were approached by pharmaceutical companies to pick herbs and plants for their products. I used to pick a range of herbs and plants, and sell them to pharmaceutical companies. This helped me to fund my education, to buy my own books and stationery to support myself through school.

Pharmaceutical companies gave us pictures of the plants and herbs they wanted picked with instructions on how to dry them. Then on the last Sunday of each month, we would bring the picked herbs and plants to school and be paid for them in cash. We were very happy to be rewarded for our work. This encouraged us to do better each time, and to pick even more herbs and plants.

Start to use fresh herbs when you are preparing your meal. Herbs are easy to grow in pots under verandahs or on balconies, they take very little space. I grow my own including: parsley, coriander, basil, thyme, rosemary, mint, chives, oregano, sage, and lemon balm. Growing herbs and spices enhances your garden, and protects your flowers and vegetables from insects. For example, planting geranium, mint and lavender at your BBQ or outdoor eating area will keep mosquitos away.

If you have a health condition or you are on medication, always consult your doctor first. Some herbs and spices may interfere with the medication that you are taking.

When you start to use herbs and spices for the first time, start with a small amount. Using herbs and spices in cooking adds extra flavour and taste to your food. It also cuts down the use of salt in cooking. At the same time, they add health benefits to you and your family.

Some herbs can be used as a whole: leaves, stalk and roots. When you have more fresh herbs than you can use, you can dry them and store them in glass jars. They keep a fresh aroma for six months. You can use herbs and spices in every dish you cook, on salads as a garnish or for extra flavour and health benefits.

When you are using dry herbs, you need to use less because they are more potent. Spices come from roots, bark and seeds.

Selection of herbs:

Basil sweet	Thai basil	Bay leaf
Chervil	Chives	Coriander
Dill	Lavender	Lemon balm
Lemon basil	Lemon thyme	Marjoram
Mint basic	Vietnamese mint	Oregano
Parsley continental (flat leaf)	Parsley curly	Rosemary
Sage	Tarragon	Thyme basic

Selection of spices:

Allspice	Black pepper	Cardamom
Caraway seeds	Cayenne pepper	Chinese five spice
Cinnamon	Cloves	Cumin
Curry powder	Fennel	Galangal
Garlic	Ginger	Lemon grass
Nutmeg	Onion, red, brown, white	Sichuan pepper
Red peppers (mild, hot very hot)	White pepper	Pink salt
Sea salt	Shallots	Spring onion
Star anise	Turmeric	

Thermogenic Spices

In the recipes below, I am using thermogenic spices that can assist your body to heal to optimal health again. They will change your taste buds, and adjust your need for fatty and sugary foods. Any time when you are preparing your meal, you can start with a small amount of these spices. As you start to develop your taste, you can increase the amount to the optimal level that is right for you.

It is best to buy spices in seeds, and to grind them in smaller quantities. Then store them in glass jars to keep the aroma and freshness for longer. It is best to grind the spices in a spice grinder, a coffee grinder or use a mortar and pestle to crush them just before cooking.

The following thermogenic spices work in synergy with each other, and are all gluten free:
- Cardamom, Cumin, Turmeric, Cayenne pepper, Caraway seeds, Fennel seeds, Smoked paprika, Fenugreek, Cinnamon, Clowes.
- Cinnamon is very good to add to coffee, porridge and apples, as it helps to balance blood sugar.

All of the above spices work synergistically together to help reduce inflammation and pain in the body. The less inflammation there is in the body, the less the potential for cancer and other illness.

Gluten free

Avoid any white flour, processed carbohydrates and sugars if you are gluten intolerant or you have coeliac disease. For people whom are gluten sensitive or intolerant, they need to look carefully for products that are 100% gluten free. Good alternatives are products from: coconut, buckwheat, brown rice, and quinoa.

Healthy Clean Food

To correct your body's balance you need to start eating healthy, clean food, free from additives, colours, preservatives, added artificial sugars, sodium/salt, fillers and thickeners. You need to get familiar with reading labels, and have handy a pocket size list of potentially dangerous substances.

When I was diagnosed with cancer, I made the decision to avoid any prepackaged food. I took time when doing the shopping so I only bought healthy and clean food. Anything that I could make, I made so that I knew what was in my food.

Rainbow of colours

Use salads and vegetables of all different colours to get all the possible nutrients in their natural form. You can eat these salads and vegetables any time of the day. Yes, even for breakfast, during any time of the year. Vegetables are good steamed slowly so they stay firm. You can find already mixed coloured salad leaves in good fruit shops and grocery stores. Or you can buy one green, one red lettuce, some rocket leaves, and fresh herbs. Then mix them all together to get a colourful salad – a rainbow of colour.

My Favourite Healthy and Nutritious Recipes

On the following pages you will find the recipes that I have created during my recovery. You may need to make adjustments to suit your needs. Any time you use any canned beans, lentils, chick peas, etc., make sure you rinse them well under cold running water before use.

1. HUMOUS DIP

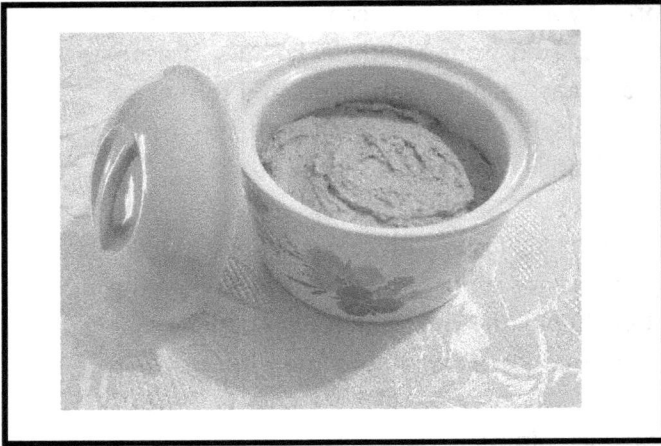

Ingredients:

200 grams of cooked or canned chick peas

1 tablespoon Tahini (unhulled)

1 teaspoon crushed garlic

1 teaspoon Moroccan spices

1 tablespoon extra-virgin cold pressed olive oil

Juice of ½ lemon

¼ teaspoon cayenne pepper

1 tablespoon chopped chives

Instructions:

1. Remove skin from the chick peas by soaking in cold alkaline water, and place the chick peas in the food processor.
2. Add all remaining ingredients, and process into a smooth paste. Add olive oil to get a spreadable texture.
3. Place the mixture in a glass bowl, cover with cling wrap, and place in refrigerator. Eat as a snack or use as a substitute for butter on bread, crackers, sandwiches, flat bread or chapati bread.

2. AVOCADO DIP

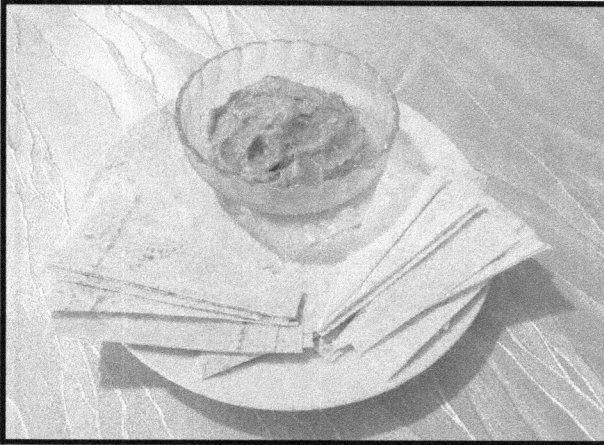

Ingredients:
- 1 very ripe avocado, healthy and without any blemishes
- Juice of one lemon
- 1 teaspoon turmeric powder

Instructions:
1. Remove skin and pip from the avocado.
2. Using a fork, mix avocado with lemon juice and turmeric powder until you have a spreadable mixture.
3. Place the mixture in a glass bowl, cover with cling wrap, and place in refrigerator. Eat as a snack or use as a substitute for butter on bread, crackers, sandwiches, flat bread or chapati bread.

Optional:
You can add natural yogurt, natural cottage cheese or goat cheese. You can also add a teaspoon of vegetable powder or spirulina.

3. CHAPATI BREAD

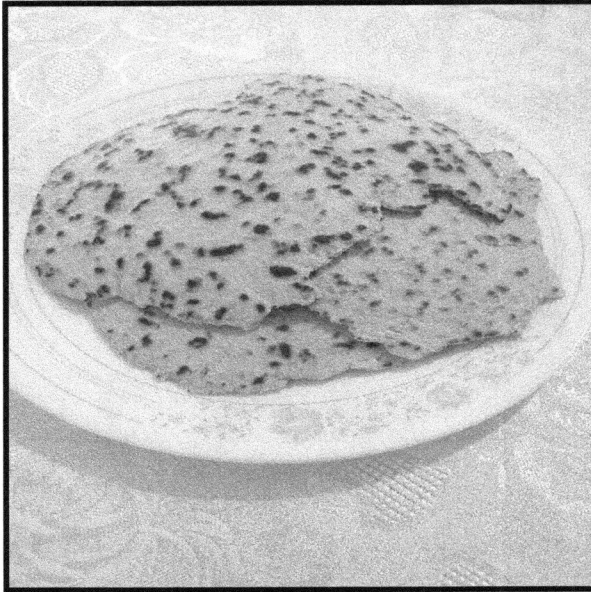

Ingredients (6 serves):
- 2 cups of flour (you can mix whole meal spelt flour, buckwheat flour, barley flour to make the 2 cup quantity)
- ½ teaspoon salt
- 4 tablespoons olive oil
- 8 tablespoons water
- 1 teaspoon minced garlic
- 1 teaspoon turmeric powder

Instructions:
1. In a medium bowl, sift all dry ingredients, add water and oil.

2. Mix the ingredients with clean hands, kneed until firm and elastic. Add extra water or olive oil if the mixture is too dry.
3. Divide into 6 balls. Roll each one as flat as possible with a rolling pin, to shape them as pancakes.
4. Smear a frying pan with a drop of oil. Heat the frying pan, medium to high.
5. Cook the chapatti on both sides until golden brown.
6. If desired, sprinkle with olive oil before serving. You can use this bread with dips or as roll ups for lunches.

4. CHICKEN SOUP

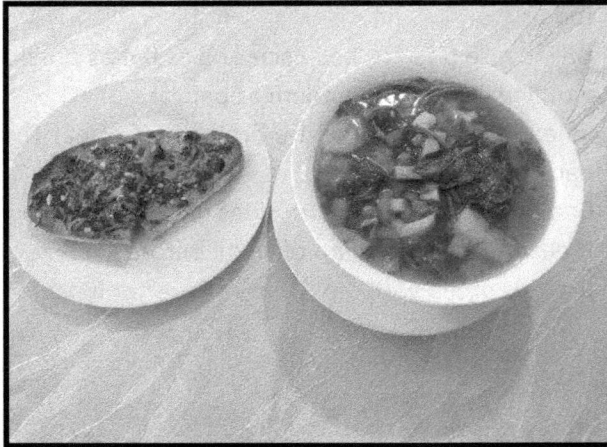

Ingredients (serves 4):

- 1 medium onion, peeled and diced
- 1 knob of ginger, finely cut
- 2 cloves of garlic, chopped
- ¼ red capsicum, chopped
- 1 litre chicken stock, prepared in advance
- 2 tablespoons olive oil
- 2 cups mixed vegetables (celery, carrots, green beans, peas), chopped/diced
- 1 bok choy/spinach leaves, washed and chopped
- Chopped parsley
- Chopped coriander
- Pinch of salt

Instructions:

1. Place oil in medium pot on medium heat. Add onion, ginger, garlic and capsicum, with a pinch of salt. Stir through until translucent.

2. Add vegetables and cook until soft.
3. Add chicken stock and stir through. Bring to boil. Add water if needed. Cover with lid.
4. After boiling for 5 minutes, add bok choy/spinach, parsley and coriander.
5. Cover and turn off the heat. Leave for 5 minutes. Serve with garlic bread.

5. SOURDOUGH TOAST WITH SPINACH, MUSHROOMS AND POACHED EGGS

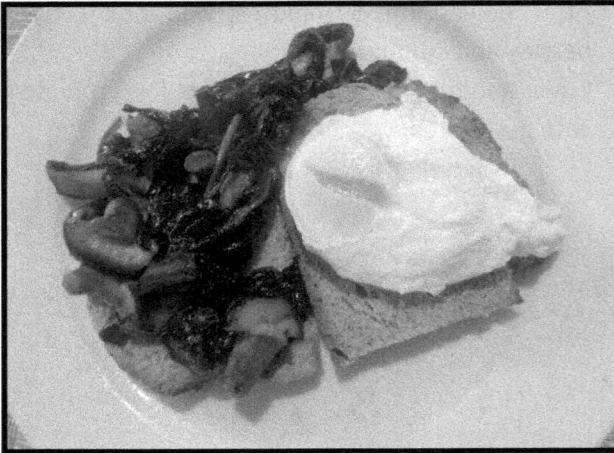

Ingredients (serves 1):
- garlic
- ginger
- spring onion
- olive oil
- mushrooms
- spinach leaves
- salt and pepper
- apple cider vinegar
- 2 eggs
- bread

Instructions:
1. Place chopped garlic, ginger, and spring onion in a frypan with olive oil. Cook for one minute, add chopped mushrooms and mix through.

2. Add spinach leaves and mix through. Season with salt and pepper.
3. To poach eggs: bring water to boil in a medium pot, add 1 tablespoon apple cider vinegar. Add one egg at a time, and let cook for 3 minutes.
4. In the meantime, toast bread.
5. Place toast on plate, top with mushrooms, spinach and eggs.

6. HEALTHY & NUTRITIOUS SUMMER SALAD

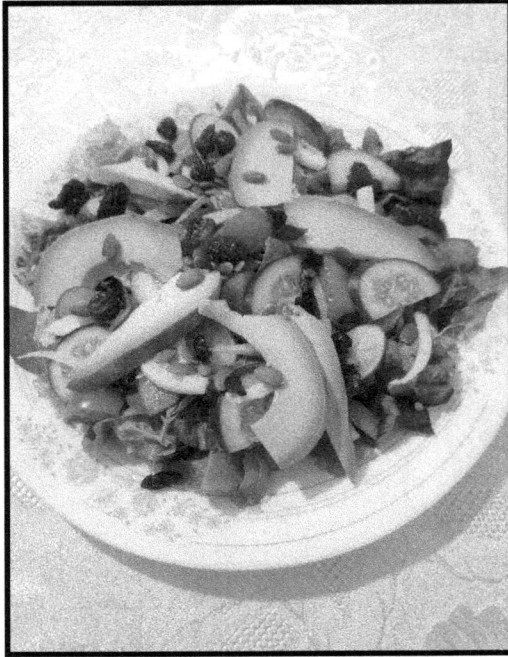

Ingredients (serves 2):
- Salad leaves
- Red and yellow peppers
- Red and yellow cherry tomatoes
- Cucumber
- Fennel
- Pepito seeds
- Sunflower seeds
- Pomegranate seeds
- Radishes
- Carrots
- Goat, feta or other soft cheese
- Grilled organic chicken or turkey breast fillet or avocado

- Steamed fresh vegetables (green beans, broccoli, asparagus, snow peas)
- Cold pressed extra virgin olive oil
- Flaxseed oil
- Lemon juice or apple cider vinegar
- Crushed garlic
- Salt, pepper

Instructions:

1. Clean and wash all salad leaves. Drain excess water, and place the leaves in a salad bowl.
2. Top the leaves with sliced red and yellow peppers, red and yellow cherry tomatoes, fresh cucumbers (leave the skin on), finely sliced fresh fennel, grated radishes and carrots.
3. Sprinkle pepito seeds, sunflower seeds, and pomegranate seeds over the top. Be creative – use any other combination that you like.
4. Add goat, feta or other soft cheese. Avoid hard processed yellow cheeses.
5. You can steam fresh vegetables, cool them and put them on top of the salad. If you plan ahead, you can add grilled organic chicken, turkey breast fillet, or avocado. Slice these on top of the salad.

Dressing:

Always make your own salad dressing. Use cold pressed extra virgin olive oil, flaxseed oil, lemon juice or apple cider vinegar, crushed garlic, salt and pepper. Combine all the ingredients, pour over the salad and mix through.

Always choose fresh ingredients that are in season and available.

7. MIXED VEGETABLES OR MIXED SALAD WITH GRILLED HALOUMI

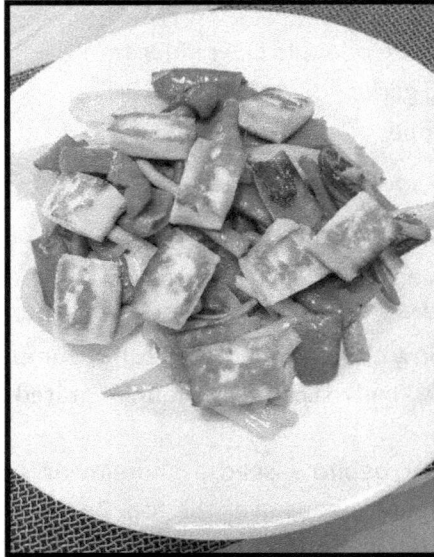

Ingredients (serves 2):
- Mixed stir-fried vegetables or salad
- 1 Haloumi, low salt
- 1 teaspoon of cold pressed extra virgin olive oil
- Salad dressing (as above)

Instructions:
1. Cook vegetables or prepare salad on a plate.
2. For the salad, prepare salad dressing.
3. Cut haloumi into 1 cm thick pieces.
4. Heat a frying pan with olive oil.
5. When the pan is heated, place haloumi pieces into the pan, and cook until golden brown on both sides.
6. Place haloumi on pre-prepared vegetables or salad. For the salad, pour dressing over the haloumi, and enjoy.

8. CHICKEN STROGONOV

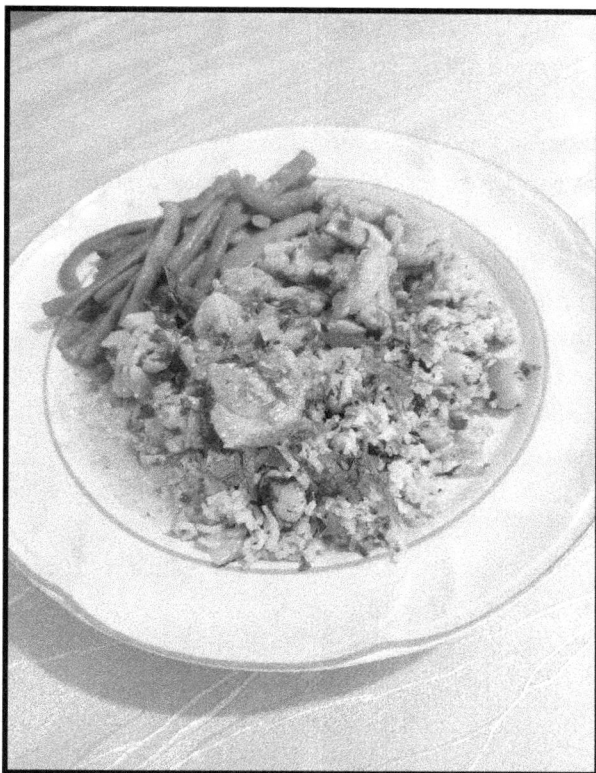

Ingredients (serves 4):
- 1 kg chicken meat, no bones
- 1 onion
- 2 cloves of garlic
- 6 button mushrooms
- ½ cup of white wine
- 1 tablespoon of sweet paprika
- 1 tablespoon tomato paste
- 500 ml. chicken stock
- 2 tablespoons of olive oil

For garnish:
- 2 tablespoons of light sour cream
- Chopped dill or parsley

Instructions:
1. Put 2 tablespoons of olive oil into a shallow pan, and heat.
2. Cut the chicken into bite size pieces. Place chicken into the pan and cook on both sides. Remove chicken from the pan and place on a side plate.
3. In the same pan add more oil and chopped onion, garlic and sliced mushrooms. Cook through. Add tomato paste and sweet paprika. Stir through.
4. Add the previously cooked chicken pieces into the pan.
5. Add wine and stir through.
6. Add stock and cook until the sauce reduces to the thickness you want.
7. Add sour cream and stir through.
8. Garnish with dill or parsley. Serve with brown rice or quinoa, and steamed green vegetables.

9. QUINOA AND HEALTHY VEGETABLES OR SALAD

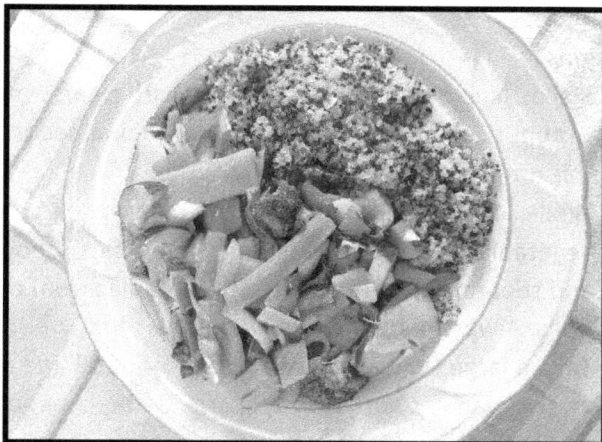

Ingredients (serves 4):

- 1 cup of quinoa
- 1 tablespoon of coconut oil
- 1 tablespoon of olive oil
- 1 medium onion
- 2 cloves of fresh garlic
- ½ cup of fresh fennel
- 1 small red pepper
- small knob of fresh ginger
- 1 teaspoon of turmeric
- sweet potato
- green leafy vegetables (broccoli, bock choy, spinach), green beans, snow peas
- juice of ½ lemon
- ½ cup of Brag's sauce
- ½ teaspoon pink salt

Quinoa is a very healthy substitute for pasta, potatoes and rice. It is important to soak it for 30 minutes in cold water, and rinse it until the water is completely clear.

Instructions:
1. Place 1 cup of quinoa in a pot, top with clean water so it is about 2 centimeters above the quinoa seeds. Cook this until all the water is evaporated.
2. While the quinoa is cooking, start to cook the vegetables. First wash all the vegetables, chop them and separate the green leaved vegetables from the hard ones. Always cook the hard vegetables first.
3. Take a large frying pan, and put coconut oil and olive oil in the pan. Chop onion, garlic, fennel, pepper and ginger.
4. Heat oils on medium heat. Cook onion, garlic, peppers, fennel, ginger, salt and turmeric. Add sweet potato and vegetables. Finish with juice of ½ lemon and Brag's sauce.
5. Serve vegetables on top of quinoa. Put any left overs in the fridge for later use. You can serve this with grilled fish, grilled chicken or cold on salad.

10.   HEALTHY PIZZA

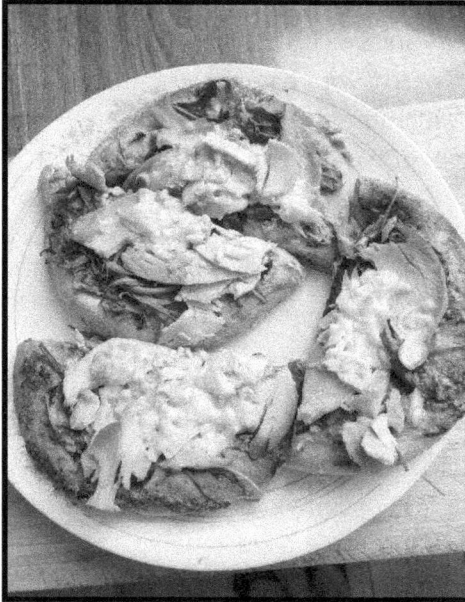

Ingredients: (serves 2)
- one sheet frozen Borgs puff pastry or pita bread or flat bread
- olive oil
- egg
- fresh goat cheese or sliced avocado
- 1 medium onion
- 2 cloves of garlic
- small knob of fresh ginger
- ½ cup of fennel, finely sliced
- 1 small sweet potato, finely sliced
- ½ cup of fresh chopped parsley, fresh coriander and basil leaves
- handful of fresh spinach

Instructions:
1. Take one sheet of frozen Borgs puff pastry, place it on a flat tray and pre-brush it with oil.
2. Brush pastry with egg and place it in the oven at 200 C for 10 minutes or until lightly brown.
3. Take it out of the oven and top with pizza topping below. Crumble fresh goat feta cheese over the top or use sliced avocado instead.
4. Pour left over egg over the pizza, and put it back into the oven for 15 minutes.
5. Remove from the over and cut the pizza into 4 slices. Serve with salad.

If you are using pita or flat bread instead of puff pastry, lightly toast one side first under a grill. Then take the pita or flat bread out of the grill and place pizza topping on the pita/flat bread. Place under grill again until cooked.

Pizza topping instructions:
1. Slice onion, garlic, ginger, fennel and sweet potato.
2. Place 1 tablespoon of olive oil into a frying pan with the above ingredients, stir fry all for 3 minutes.
3. Add fresh chopped parsley, fresh coriander, basil leaves and handful of fresh spinach. Now you have the topping ready for your pizza.

11. PULSE PASTA

This pasta is rich in protein, is a very good substitute for meat and is easy to make.

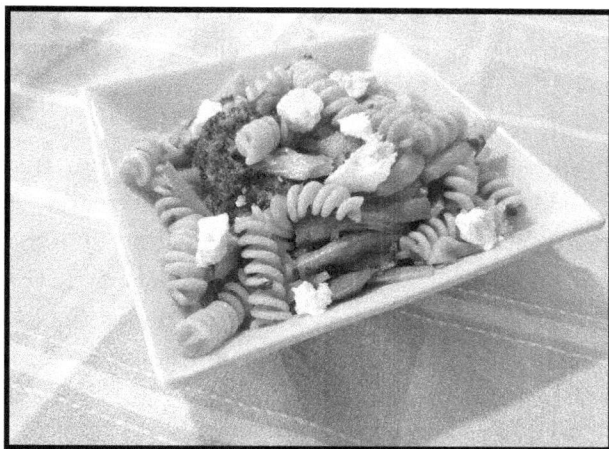

Ingredients (serves 2):

- 2 cups of dry Pulse pasta
- 1 teaspoon of salt
- 1 tablespoon olive oil
- 1 medium onion
- ½ red pepper
- 1 clove fresh garlic
- knob of fresh ginger
- Any vegetables in season of your choice
- Spices of your choice
- Soft cheese of your choice

Instructions:
1. Boil water in a pot, add salt to water once it boils.
2. Add dry pasta to boiling water, and cook until almost soft.
3. While the pasta is cooking, add 1 tablespoon olive oil in a frying pan and start to prepare the vegetables.
4. Chop onion, pepper, garlic, ginger and add spices of your choice. Place in hot frypan and cook until all are soft, avoid burning.
5. When cooked, add pasta to the same frying pan.
6. Add a handful of spinach leaves, shredded kale or vegetables of your choice. Stir together until the leaves are wilted or the vegetables are cooked. If you need, add some of the pasta water to make the sauce.
7. Serve with soft cheese of your choice. Creamy goat cheese is a good option.

12. GRILLED SALMON WITH MIXED SALAD OR STIR-FRIED VEGETABLES

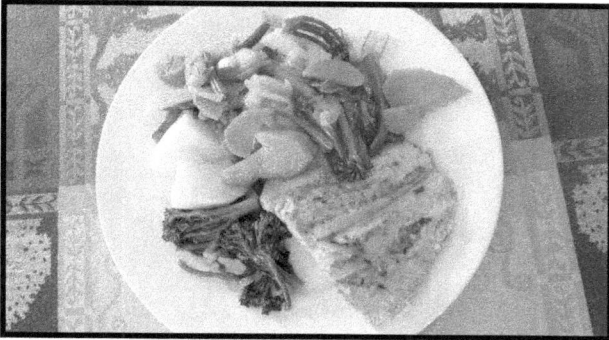

Ingredients (serves 1):

- Fresh salmon
- Lemon
- Sea salt
- Moroccan spices

Instructions:

1. Marinate salmon with lemon, sea salt, and Moroccan spices. Leave it to sit for 10 minutes at room temperature.
2. Heat a frypan with olive oil.
3. Cook the salmon with skin down for 2 to 3 minutes, turn over and cook for 2 minutes on other side.
4. Serve with pre-prepared salad or vegetables.

13. COCOA PUFF SLICES (no cooking required)

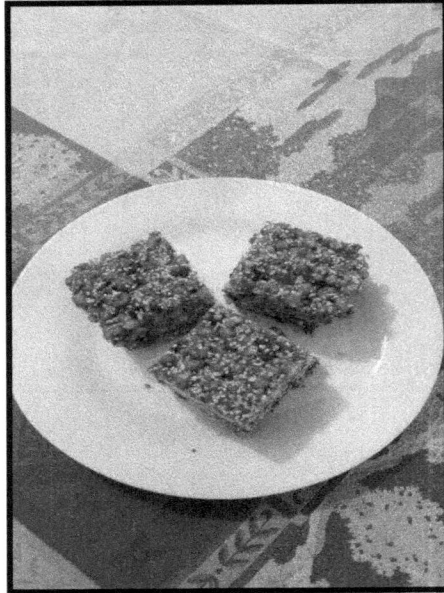

Dry Ingredients:
- 3 cups of brown rice puffs
- ½ cup of chia seeds
- ½ cup of sesame seeds
- 1 heaped teaspoon of turmeric powder
- 3 heaped teaspoons of cocoa powder
- ½ cup of dried currants
- ½ cup of dried cranberries
- ½ cup of shredded coconut
- ½ teaspoon of pink salt
- 3 teaspoons of cinnamon
- ½ cup of LSA

Wet Ingredients:
- 60 ml of rice malt syrup
- 60 ml of coconut oil
- 1/3 cup of boiling water

Instructions for 16 slices:
1. In a large bowl, place all the dry ingredients.
2. In a small bowl, mix all the wet ingredients. Combine well into a liquid.
3. Using a fork, combine dry and wet ingredients together in the large bowl. Make sure that it is well combined - if it is too dry, add hot water as needed.
4. Line a 20 x 20 cm square dish with baking paper, including the sides of the dish.
5. Slowly pour the mixture into the dish. Using a spatula, press the mixture firmly in the corners and sides of the dish. Make sure the top of the mixture is nice and flat. Cover the dish with cling wrap, and place it in the fridge overnight.
6. Using a sharp knife, cut the puffs into equal size squares to make 16 slices. Place in an air tight container, and keep it in the fridge. These are great for snacks or lunchboxes.

14. BANANA MUFFINS or BANANA SLICES

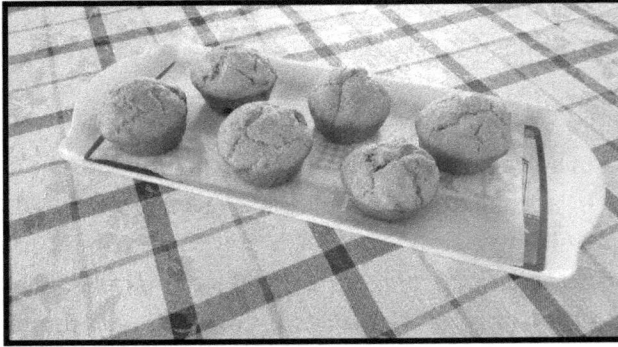

Dry Ingredients:
- 1 cup of almond meal
- 1/3 cup of quick cook oats
- 1/3 cup of chopped cashews or walnuts
- ½ teaspoon of baking powder
- 1 teaspoon of cinnamon
- ½ teaspoon of turmeric powder
- Pinch of salt

Wet Ingredients:
- 1½ small or 1 large ripe banana, mashed with a fork
- 1/3 cup of almond milk
- ¼ cup of melted coconut oil
- 1 egg

Instructions for 12 muffins:
1. In a large bowl, mix all dry ingredients. Combine well.
2. In a small bowl, mix all wet ingredients. Combine well.
3. Pour the wet ingredients into the dry ones, and combine well.

4. Line a muffin baking dish with 2 strips of baking paper for each muffin mould. Place the baking strips across each other to form a cross. Using a spoon, pour the mixture evenly into the baking dish. Then sprinkle each muffin with chopped nuts.
5. Bake until nice and brown. Bake in the oven at 180 C for approximately 25 minutes or until the tester is dry.
6. Cool muffins/slices on a rack. Ideal for morning tea or in lunch boxes.

For slices:

If you want to make slices instead, you can make double the amount of mixture. Then line a 20 x 20 cm baking dish with baking paper, pour the mixture into the dish making sure it is level on top. Bake for about 45 minutes.

15. CINNAMON OAT AND WALNUT COOKIES

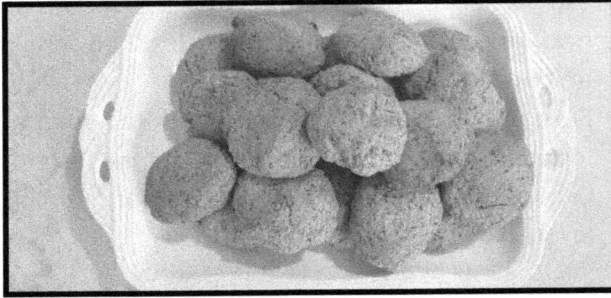

Ingredients (makes 16 cookies):

- 1 ½ cups whole meal flour
- 2 tablespoons brown sugar
- 1 cup of Australian oats
- 1 cup of walnut pieces
- ½ cup buttermilk
- ¼ cup melted butter
- 1 teaspoon cinnamon
- ½ teaspoon bicarb soda
- 1 teaspoon salt

Instructions:

1. Preheat the oven to 175 Celsius. Line a baking tray with baking paper.
2. Add all ingredients to a food processor, and blitz together until they form a dough consistency.
3. Roll 2 tablespoons of the dough mixture into a ball. Repeat until you have used all the dough. Place balls on the lined baking tray.
4. Bake for 15-20 minutes. Cool and enjoy.

How to repair your gut health

On a daily basis we need to eat food that is rich in prebiotics to balance out good and bad gut bacteria. If you are on medication or are having constant gut problems, you must repair your gut.

Before each meal take 1 to 2 tablespoons of fermented food such as: natural yogurt, Kiefer, Kombucha, Sauerkraut. Look for Sauerkraut that is made with salt and water only. Buy it in glass jars only. Start with a small amount, and slowly increase the amount until your reach the amount that you are comfortable with.

Here is my personal recipe for a salad that you can eat before any meal.

1. Take a large glass bowl. In it place 500 grams of sauerkraut, a medium carrot grated, medium red onion grated, 2 small cloves of fresh garlic grated, 1 tablespoon of fresh ginger grated, 1 cup fresh fennel grated, ½ cup fresh parsley chopped, 1 small red apple grated, 1 teaspoon cumin seeds, 1 teaspoon pink salt and ½ cup cold pressed olive oil.
2. Mix all the ingredients well with your hands. Cover with glad wrap, and place in the fridge.

Eat ½ cup before each meal or place a good handful of fresh spinach leaves on the plate, and top with the mixture. Enjoy as a meal, and place left overs back in the fridge.

For more details on gut health, please refer to Chpter 12 of this book.

I hope that the information and recipes in this book help you to create better health for you and your family. I am also hoping that I have achieved my outcome by writing this book, of helping to empower every reader as to how to gain and maintain optimal health.

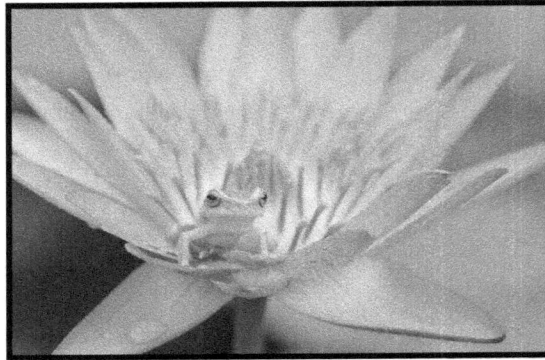

Appendix

Additional Resources to Empower You for Optimal Body-Mind Health

- If you have any **questions** about transforming your mindset, emotions, beliefs, self-doubts, stress, habits and health, please email Dr Vesna Grubacevic at vesna@qttransformation.com
- Visit **www.qttransformation.com** for:
- **your free resources** to empower yourself for greater confidence, health and success
- **Stop Sabotaging Your Confidence book**: your step-by-step workbook filled with simple and effective techniques that you can apply to transform self-sabotage into lasting confidence and success.
- **Quickly, easily and permanently free yourself** from your fears, anxieties, trauma, stress, bad habits, self-sabotage and negative/toxic personal and professional relationships... and create a great relationship, a fulfilling career and an abundance of confidence, success, health and happiness
- **Unhappy in your career? Looking for a career change? Love helping people?** Experience your own personal transformation, learn 100s of amazing techniques to help others, and retrain as a successful, skilled and confident Hypnotherapist, NLP and Qt respect i® Practitioner, and make a difference to others' lives. Join Dr Vesna on this rewarding journey.
- For enquiries about our scholarships, please email info@qttransformation.com

Other Health Resources

- "The Shopping Guide" and "The Chemical Maze", by Bill Stathman
- "What Your Doctor May Not Tell You, May Kill You", by Dr. John Lee
- "The Human Body: How We Fail, How We Heal", by Professor Anthony A. Goodman
- "Stay Young and Sexy with Bio-Identical Hormone Replacement", by Dr. Jonatan V. White and Lane Lenard PhD.
- "The Acid & Alkaline Food Guide", by Dr, Susan E. Brown and Larry Trivieri, Jr.
- "Balancing Body Chemistry", by Michael Cutler, MD
- "Raw Juices Can Save Your Life", by Dr. Sandra Cabot
- "No Guts, No Glory", by Steven Lamm, MD and Sidney Stevens
- "The Role of Herbs and Spices in Cancer Prevention", by Christine M Kaefer et al., Journal of Nutritional Biochemistry June 2008.
- Dr. Rath Research Institute https://www.drrathresearch.org/
- www.digestivehealth.com.au
- www.cancerscreening.gov.au
- www.breastscreen.org.au
- www.jeanhailes.org.au

Nevenka's Upcoming Book

How I survived a male dominated world and bullying for over 50 years

Chapter 1 References:

Grubacevic, PhD, Vesna, Stop Sabotaging Your Confidence: How to Transform Self Sabotage into Lasting Confidence and Success, Melbourne: Vesna Corporation Pty Ltd, 2014, pp 3-4, 95, Chapters 3, 4 & 9.

Chopra, MD., Deepak, Quantum Healing: Exploring the Frontiers of Mind/Body Medicine, New York: Bantam Books, 1989, pp. 54-55

Gordon EM, Chauvin RJ, Van AN, Rajesh A, Nielsen A, Newbold DJ, Lynch CJ, Seider NA, Krimmel SR, Scheidter KM, Monk J, Miller RL, Metoki A, Montez DF, Zheng A, Elbau I, Madison T, Nishino T, Myers MJ, Kaplan S, Badke D'Andrea C, Demeter DV, Feigelis M, Ramirez JSB, Xu T, Barch DM, Smyser CD, Rogers CE, Zimmermann J, Botteron KN, Pruett JR, Willie JT, Brunner P, Shimony JS, Kay BP, Marek S, Norris SA, Gratton C, Sylvester CM, Power JD, Liston C, Greene DJ, Roland JL, Petersen SE, Raichle ME, Laumann TO, Fair DA, Dosenbach NUF. A Somato-Cognitive Action Network alternates with effector regions in motor cortex. Nature. April 19, 2023. DOI: 10.1038/s41586-023-05964-2

E. Mostofsky, E. A. Penner, M. A. Mittleman. Outbursts of anger as a trigger of acute cardiovascular events: a systematic review and meta-analysis. *European Heart Journal*, 2014; DOI: 10.1093/eurheartj/ehu033

Haase, Claudia M.; Holley, Sarah; Bloch, Lian; Verstaen, Alice; Levenson, Robert W. Interpersonal Emotional Behaviors and Physical Health: A 20-Year Longitudinal Study of Long-Term Married Couples. *Emotion*, 2016 DOI: 10.1037/a0040239

Watson, Beyond Supernature, pp.58-60

Keith Petrie and John Weinman. Patients' Perceptions of Their Illness: The Dynamo of Volition in Health Care. *Current Directions in Psychological Science*, 2012

Siani, L. M., Dr., "The Link Between Stress and Illness", *Access*, Journal of the ABH and ABNLP, Spring 2003, p. 4

https://www.medicalnewstoday.com/articles/stress-vs-anxiety#when-to-see-a-doctor

Lipton, B.H., The Biology of Belief, Unleashing the Power of Consciousness, Matter and Miracles, Hay House Inc, USA, 2008, p. 43

Cancer Council Victoria website, Family History and Cancer, https://www.cancervic.org.au/cancer-information/genetics-and-risk/family-history-of-cancer

Chapter 11 Reference:

https://fluoridealert.org/articles/50-reasons/   includes   an abundance of research and studies on fluoride.

Chapter 12 Reference:

Jessica D. Hathaway-Schrader, Heidi M. Steinkamp, Michael B. Chavez, Nicole A. Poulides, Joy E. Kirkpatrick, Michael E. Chew, Emily Huang, Alexander V. Alekseyenko, Jose I. Aguirre, Chad M. Novince. Antibiotic Perturbation of Gut Microbiota Dysregulates Osteoimmune Cross Talk in Postpubertal Skeletal Development. *The American Journal of Pathology*, 2019.

About the Authors

Nevenka Malic

Nevenka was a highly passionate, driven and dedicated professional. Her strong ethic is reflected in her clients' success. Her excellent communication skills and deep understanding of nutrition, food and health assist Nevenka to simply and effectively explain even the most complex concepts to her clients.

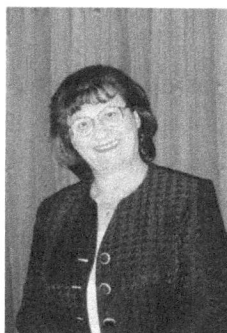

Her philosophy is that nutrition plays an important component in the recovery of any health issue. Nevenka strongly believes in going back to basics, and drawing on the wisdom of how food has been prepared by our ancestors. The more natural the food we eat, the better the chance that the body can recover. Nevenka believes that food is our medicine, and she works on a deeper level to address the whole body-mind to help people achieve optimal long-term health.

A firm supporter of prevention, Nevenka focuses on keeping the body healthy before it breaks down. She always begins with good quality fresh food then supplements as needed. Every single body is different especially if the person has any health conditions. Therefore, she assesses each individual before designing their individual program. Nevenka empowers her clients with the self-belief, skills and knowledge so that they can sustain the successes they achieve with her, in the long term.

Nevenka believes that every person deserves a second chance to be healthy and happy. Having been through many personal and health challenges in her own life, Nevenka has adapted to life changes many times, and is very familiar with the difficulties that accompany these.

A history of serious illness and injuries gave Nevenka a determination to heal herself. She set off on her healing journey, re-educating herself in a healthier lifestyle. By using complimentary therapies, in combination with a nutritional and healthy eating plan, she has seen outstanding results. As a cancer survivor, Nevenka is also passionate about assisting others to deal with the recovery process after major life changing conditions.

Professional Experience

Nevenka's life has revolved around people, food, health and business. She grew up on a farm in Europe and has from an early age been exposed to growing organic produce, cooking and using nature for healing as taught by her grandmother. With those solid foundations, Nevenka then spent the next 40 years combining her love of food, people, health and business in the hospitality industry, both overseas and in Australia. For over 10 years, Nevenka also ran a very successful restaurant, managing dozens of employees to deliver great food and customer experience.

She has also researched food and environmental health for over 20 years and has worked with numerous clients over that time, developing and using a unique combination of techniques to achieve outstanding results with them.

Nevenka has contributed her cooking skills and presented at the Slow Cooking Festival at Federation Square. She has also been invited to contribute articles and recipes to the book "Thank you Mum", a tribute to European and Middle Eastern migrants who have contributed to Melbourne's cuisine. Nevenka also presented and educated on healthy cooking at the Multicultural Society. She has also taught cooking and baking at community centres, and gluten free cooking at Celiac and Food Intolerance groups.

With a unique background and experience in nutrition and gastronomy, Nevenka helps people to know exactly what they need to eat for their own nutrition and health recovery, as well as teaches them how to prepare healthy nutritious meals in less than 20 minutes.

Nevenka's qualifications include

Bachelor of Hotel Management (obtained in Europe) and qualified Chef
Diploma in Clinical Nutrition
Diploma in Food and Environmental Allergies
Advanced Aromatic Manual Lymphatic Drainage
Certified Reiki Master Practitioner
Head, Neck and Shoulder Massage
Crystal Healing Therapist
Infrabed Thermal Therapy
Certified Advanced Clinical Hypnotherapist, Master NLP Practitioner and Qt respect i® Practitioner

Dr Vesna Grubacevic

Dr. Vesna Grubacevic is driven by making a profound difference, and has dedicated her life to empowering others. She is the founder of multi award-winning company Qt, Performance Transformation Expert®, an internationally recognised and Certified NLP and Hypnotherapy Trainer, Qt respect i® Creator and Certified Trainer, Advanced Clinical Hypnotherapist, and Master NLP Practitioner.

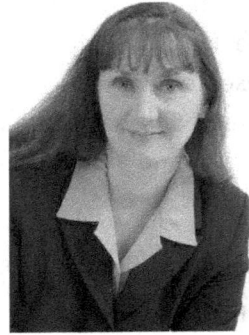

She also holds a PhD, a BEc, is the author of *Stop Sabotaging Your Confidence* best-selling book, and the Transformational NLP Guide, co-author of *Game Changers: Innovation in Business*, creator of the *Self Empowerment Technique©,* is a passionate speaker, and multi award-winning leader and innovator in her field.

With well over 41 years of experience in business (including in economics, domestic and international financial markets, global strategy, cultural change in multinational organisations, hospitality, and working with CEOs, executives, professionals, salespeople, business owners, managers, teams and individuals), Dr. Vesna has mastered the art and science of understanding behaviour and performance on an individual, business, organisational, economy wide and global level.

Her diversity of experience with corporations, business, health, spirituality and the arts enables Dr. Vesna to understand, relate easily and be in tune with people from any field. This diversity of training experience, fun, passion and innate ability to simply, effectively and clearly communicate the most complex of concepts makes her unique in the field.

She founded Qt in 2000, driven by her vision to create an empowered society. Since then, she has run numerous NLP/Hypnotherapy/Qt respect i® certification trainings and trained and certified many successful practitioners (including coaches, therapists, medical, allied health and mental health practitioners, managers, business owners and leaders) so they too can empower others.

Dr. Vesna has also worked with thousands of individuals and professionals to transform their personal and professional success, as well as assisted businesses to transform their individual, team and leadership performance and business culture.

Through her PhD research, further studies and experience in successfully working with thousands of clients, Dr Vesna also developed Qt respect i®, innovative advanced behavioural change techniques. After working with many clients and identifying a gap in the market and an unmet client need, Dr. Vesna created these unique multi-award winning, transformational techniques. Finally, there is now a proven, safe and recognised way to permanently stop the disempowering dynamics with other people and get the respect, love and appreciation you deserve!

Dr. Vesna's passion for transformation and empowering others to excel both personally and professionally is reflected in the exceptional results she achieves with her clients. Often described by her clients, colleagues and friends as having the highest levels of integrity, professionalism, ethics and congruence, Dr. Vesna lives and breathes all that she teaches. Her drive for excellence and dedication to her clients is reflected in her proven track record of empowering clients to achieve exceptional personal and professional results, fast.

Having had many challenges in her life, both personally and professionally, Dr. Vesna has been through her own personal transformation journey - from decades of being bullied and being in toxic personal and professional relationships, she has transformed her confidence, relationships and herself to being a confident and successful business owner. To empower others on their journey, she also draws on her experience and her personal transformation journey, and inspires others to quickly transform their mindset, confidence, health, relationships and success, and to exceed their potential.

Visit www.qttransformation.com for your free resources, and empower yourself today.

Qt, Qt respect i®, respect i®, Qt 7 Secrets to Transformation®, Qt Transform Your Destiny®, and Qt Performance Transformation Expert® are all registered trademarks of Vesna Corporation Pty Ltd.

www.ingramcontent.com/pod-product-compliance
Lightning Source LLC
Chambersburg PA
CBHW070922270326
41927CB00011B/2682